PRAISE FOR MALACHY: A FATHER'S STORY OF LOVE, LAUGHTER AND LOSS

The beautiful boy staring out from the book cover was sunshine itself.

I was lucky to meet Malachy in an all too familiar setting for Maggie and Dom, at Sydney's Westmead hospital. Malachy stole your heart in an instant. He'd be very proud of his Dad and his family, who have crafted an exquisite tribute to his remarkable life. With an eloquence and insight that comes in part from overwhelming pain and loss, Dom has written a book that speaks to all the complexities of the human experience. This is so much more than a guidebook to being the parents of a Heartkid; it's a deeply profound memoir about the meaning of life.

In his life, Malachy bestowed his special gifts on everyone who knew him. With this magnificent book, Dom conveys the Malachy magic to all, reminding us again that we can never take a single day for granted.

—Simon Reeve, television presenter, journalist, podcaster and HeartKids Ambassador

All around us, though we don't always know it, are parents whose children are not well. Who have anguish and grief mixed with the normal travails of raising a child. Some of these parents become able to rise up through that and muster an extra lovingness that means a hard life, or a tragically short life, can still be a beautiful one. Suffering doesn't have to break us. It can teach us to love. A beautifully written book about a beautifully loved child: this family did something special under huge stress, and we can all take heart from it.

—Steve Biddulph AM, bestselling parenting author whose books include *Manhood*, *Fully Human* and *Raising Boys*

A beautiful book and an eye-opener for all of us involved in the care of children with heart problems. Always well-intentioned but often messy, their story is a good reminder of how we can improve. Dom and Maggie's relationship with Malachy, and their investment of precious time in the development of HeartKids, both have interesting back stories.

Their loss is enormous. Dom's thoughtful humanity shines as a guiding light throughout.

—David Winlaw, Professor of Surgery, cardiothoracic surgeon, researcher, Cincinnati Children's Hospital Medical Center

Dominic Frawley's loving elegy to his cherished son is deeply moving. It is a beautiful celebration of young Malachy's life and the family who adored him. As it moves from heart-warming to heart-rending ... to heart-wrenching, there are also moments where you will laugh out loud. ('They're crying! Get the social worker!' had me chortling and smiling for some time.) Ultimately, *Malachy* is a supremely uplifting story of an irrepressible soul, beloved forever and immortalised in this tribute.

—Cindy Pan, medical practitioner, bestselling author, media personality

Joy and grief, philosophy and faith, and the everlasting bond between father and son. Through one life, Frawley explores the things that make us — and almost break us.

—Allison Tait (A.L. Tait), bestselling author middle-grade adventure series *The Mapmaker Chronicles* and the *Ateban Cipher*, and her new novel *The Fire Star*

Malachy: A father's story of love, laughter and loss is an unforgettable experience. Dom's sensitive and gifted writing style engaged me from the very beginning so that I felt as if I was involved heart and soul in the journey of Malachy's lifetime. The family dynamic that was created by six intelligent, creative, generous, loving and adventurous people enabled Malachy to achieve his potential as a human being for fourteen plus years; to pack into those years more quality of life than many folk do if they live to be a hundred. Dom enables the reader to experience his son undefended, to see the world through his eyes, so I feel as if I know him, and as if I know his beautiful family.

'Words are our tools of resurrection' is a quote I love from a character in a book by Pip Williams, *The Dictionary of Lost Words*. Dom has used his words of love, loss and grief beautifully to do just that – to bring Malachy back into life again, into his life, and into the lives of everyone who has the courage to fully experience this touching tribute to a precious son.

—Dianne McKissock OAM, sociologist, relationship counsellor, and grief therapist, Co-Founder and Patron of the Bereavement Care Centre and the National Centre for Childhood Grief, author of *Coping with Grief*

This is a very interesting book. It details the very close relationship between a father and son, perhaps intensified by the fact that Malachy had a major cardiac anomaly. On that level it provides an insight into the effect of a major illness on a family and the interactions that result from that. On another level however it clarifies the impact of a serious cardiac condition on the child and his place in the world.

While only a very small percentage of children with heart conditions are affected in this way, I think this book informs both the medical community and the patient group on this interaction and provides a very valuable insight into the effect of severe heart disease on the child, the family and his community. From my point of view it clarifies aspects of the doctor/patient relationship from the patient's perspective: an area that undoubtedly warrants further examination!

This is a "must read" for all medical professionals looking after patients like Malachy. It is likely to be of interest to other parents of children with severe cardiac conditions and particularly to potential parents in whom a cardiac condition has been identified antenatally. I would hope that a book like this enables us to improve our support of such families through a journey that at times can be extremely difficult.

—Stephen Cooper, paediatric cardiologist

MALACHY

*A father's story of love,
laughter and loss*

DOMINIC FRAWLEY

WILD
DINGO
PRESS

Published by Wild Dingo Press
Melbourne, Australia
books@wilddingopress.com.au
www.wilddingopress.com.au

First published by Wild Dingo Press 2021

Cover designer: Debra Billson
Editors: Catherine Lewis and Elise Menzies
Printed in Australia.

Frawley, Dominic 1966- author.
Malachy: A father's story of love, laughter and loss/Dominic Frawley.

A catalogue record for this
book is available from the
NATIONAL
LIBRARY   National Library of Australia
OF AUSTRALIA

ISBN: 9781925893656 (paperback)
ISBN: 9781925893663 (ebook:pdf)
ISBN: 9781925893670 (ebook)

For and with Malachy, age fourteen.
He wanted to publish his first book by fifteen.

Contents

MAGGIE'S DREAM

Such is the life of a man. Moments of joy, obliterated by unforgettable sadness. There's no need to tell the children that.

— Marcel Pagnol

Organised chaos surrounds me at my desk. The familiarity of my personal mess is a comfort to me, as my gaze settles on the neighbour's camphor laurel tree. I am thinking about my family. At 49 years of age I am making the standard adjustments every parent makes to the emptying of my family nest. My children have each forged their own futures. There is only one thing, one moment I would change.

Sometimes I want the world to stop, but not as desperately as I once did, and not for such long periods of time. People who have children believe the children make them happy. My elder daughter, Imogen, likes to remind me that the studies tell a different story. The childless report higher happiness scores on average than their fertile peers.

I try not to feel bleak. Against the evidence of my own experience, I believe happiness lies in our deepest bonds. Maggie, my wife, had this dream of our children last night:

A musty aromatic spice floats in the humid air of the restaurant. Bland cover versions of once popular tunes mingle with the scattered voices of the diners, whose cutlery clinks against patterned ceramic bowls.

Dark red carpet seems to suck the ambient light issuing from a handful of Chinese lanterns, providing dull illumination for the quiet dinnertime crowd. At one table, a mother and three children are playing out a familiar family scene. The four of them are playing our family 'question game', designed to

1

occupy and entertain the children while our food is prepared. Each person takes a turn at posing a bespoke trivia question to each of their dinner companions. Usually, the parents build learning points into their questions.

Maggie, dressed in her usual flowing, post-hippie style, is smiling. Laughter breaks out intermittently as the familial banter shifts back and forth. Her unfurrowed brow moves to engage each child in turn.

On Maggie's left is a slender, fair little girl. White-blonde hair sits neatly at the nape of her neck as she cranes energetically forward, eyes wide. This is Niamh, who in the dream looks six years old. As Maggie speaks, the little girl's eyebrows jump with surprise, her mouth forms an 'O', excitement plain to see.

An olive-skinned boy of eight murmurs something, drawing Maggie's attention to the next seat at the table, as the waitress delivers a bowl of steamed dim sims. Loose brown curls frame a cheeky grin as with one eye cocked, the boy focuses on his mother. This eight-year-old is Seamus. Maggie holds his attention, clearly the conversation is riveting to him too. Seamus's mouth drops open as his sister's had only seconds ago. Jokes spill across the table while the dinner progresses.

As Niamh and Seamus sit back to enjoy reflecting on Maggie's questions there is a brief lull in the conversation. The scene moves to the other diner, the smallest of them, lighter in colour than his brother, finely shaped like his sister. Malachy is bursting with animation and grinning widely. There is a blue tinge to his four-year-old lips as he laughs and enjoys whatever amazing revelations his mother is making.

Having left the older two to their ruminations, Maggie is now merrily focused on Malachy. His delight is palpable, pushing his way onto Mum's knee, ever one for physical contact. Dishevelled locks of light brown hair, with touches of blonde and ginger, fall this way and that. Spare shoulders hunch forward under his T-shirt. The pre-school child confidently stares up at Maggie, utters something to draw

> laughter and waits for her rejoinder. Maggie begins to speak, but falters. Puzzled, she starts again. The children's faces turn blank. Silence descends. The dream vanishes.

I jolted awake as Maggie's sobs cut through the night. I was barely asleep anyway, nursing my own sorrows through the dark of the early hours. Shaken by Maggie's sudden distress it took me a few seconds to realise what was going on.

'I'm here, Maggie.' I waited.

'I've had the worst dream,' Maggie groaned.

'Do you want to tell me about it?'

In the bedside light Maggie looked gaunt and expressionless. We caught eyes, no doubt my stare every bit as hollow as hers.

'I was at the Chinese restaurant, with the children. Just the little three. You and Imogen weren't there. I felt so happy. They were little again. We were at Nowra Palace.'

Pausing, Maggie inhaled.

'So, I was talking to them, and I realised they were younger, but I wasn't. So, it dawned on me I was back in time and they'd be keen to hear about the future.'

> 'Guys, this is cool, do you get it? I am nearly 50, but you're still young, so I can tell you about the future.'

'Of course, they wanted to know all sorts of things, so I was filling them in. I started with Niamh.'

> 'Niamh, you're growing up heaps. You're at boarding school in Sydney. You're doing your HSC, darling. You're taller than me, with long blond hair. You're still a beautiful runner. You like music and art. You're planning to go off to uni next year.'

> It was exciting. We were all excited because I knew all this stuff they hadn't been through yet. Then I told Seamus: 'Seamus, you're all grown up. You're 20, and as tall as Dom. You've got a huge mop of hair! You're at uni already. You're studying medicine, and you live in Sydney with Imogen. You've got some really great friends.'

Another pause, another breath, deep, and a shake of her head.

'I told them how I teach at St John's now, and that they all went to school there for a while, and that you're still working down the road, and we still live in Nowra. It was so lovely being back in that time.

> I felt so happy. Then Malachy was being all cute and quirky, and of course he asked me about himself. I started telling him: 'Malachy, you're getting so tall, too; you go to high school and your hair is getting a bit curly. You've been learning the drums. You love to write and ... you catch the bus, you even have your own YouTube channel ... and—'

'Then in the dream I remembered what had happened. I couldn't tell them. I realised what had happened, and I froze. Something was wrong. That's when I woke up. I couldn't tell them. I couldn't tell Malachy.'

Our hands clutching, we stared at the ceiling in the semi-darkness of our bedroom. No further words were needed.

I know, and Maggie knows, what it was in her dream. What it was she couldn't tell the children.

PART 1

INFANCY

the primordial soup

1

AN ULTRASOUND

We do not remember days. We remember moments.

— Cesare Pavese

Malachy is an Irish name, derived from the Hebrew, Malachi: Messenger of God. If our son Malachy had a message from above, we were destined to have a hard time deciphering just what it was. 'What if?' was a question he would pose time and time again, starting months before his birth.

Maggie had a routine ultrasound test 19 weeks into her fourth pregnancy. To this point, ultrasound had been a reliable source of good news in our family. The first glimpse of reproduced life in utero always has an air of the miraculous about it.

Ultrasound technology had been in rapid evolution through my lifetime. It was first used to look at human organs in the late 1940s, including the heart in the 1950s, then in the 1960s for measurement of foetal skulls during pregnancy. Constant progress had spread the technology around the world, including into the loungeroom of my childhood home. I remember as a child in the 1970s marvelling when my father, a vascular surgeon, had demonstrated a portable 'Pencil Doppler' on the artery in my wrist. He told me his 'toy' was the first such device imported into Australia. I was intrigued by his explanation that this pen-like appliance bounced sound waves into my body to measure the rush of blood through my vessels.

The very first pregnancy ultrasound I ever saw was part of my medical studies in the 1980s. At that point in history the images were still rudimentary. The grainy pictures relied more on scientific interpretation than keen eyesight. A faint blur near some leg-like shadows was used to guess the gender of the foetus. A fluttering orb in the foetal chest confirmed a heartbeat.

My second ultrasound experience arrived during Maggie's gestation of our eldest child, Imogen. I vividly recall the first moment, in 1993, when Imogen's heartbeat was transmitted into the sterile air of a consulting room in North Sydney. Maggie and I were startled to hear her tiny heart racing along, with a loud rushing sound bouncing around the room. Maggie nearly leapt from the couch as this new life burst from theory into reality. It was only in that moment that we truly believed that the delay in Maggie's cycle, and the faint blue line on a pregnancy test kit, really was a new, separate, life within.

As Maggie and I moved through the 1990s, having four babies along the way, the ultrasound pictures grew clearer with each successive pregnancy.

Ultrasound number three belongs to Seamus. Now experienced parents, we were less startled by the images, but as with Imogen's earlier study, the ultrasound for Seamus led to a bout of self-congratulation.

After Seamus was Niamh. Her foetal ultrasound, number four in my experience, ran to plan. The full range of views and measurements were hastily ticked off in a darkened room. Once more Maggie and I confirmed our great fecundity and revelled in the perfection of another delicate, prized offspring.

By 1998, so much detail could be assessed in the hands of the right operator, that all manner of malformations and anomalies, speeds of growth, and volumes of fluid and tissue could be assessed and recorded. We had even had the joy of recognising facial features in our unborn children or imagining a slight wave of the hand or curling of the upper lip to 'smile for the camera'.

In the spring of 1998, Maggie and I attended Malachy's ultrasound with an air of complacent affability. After our previous successes there was hardly a thought given to anything but the miraculous nature of human reproduction. Mother Nature seemed very adept in the manufacture and production of our babies. Professional murmurs about normal organs and correct counts of fingers and toes were the familiar background music of ultrasonography. We knew the antenatal routine: pokes and prods, then reassurance, followed by celebration.

After introductions Maggie mounted the bed. The ambient light was dimmed, and a dollop of clear jelly was squirted onto her maternally swollen tummy. She wriggled slightly—it's always a bit colder than expected. With practised skill, and just the necessary amount of small talk, the sonographer went about her intimate work. A smooth transducer was pressed against Maggie's skin, bouncing its sound waves in to throw images onto the screen. Here are the legs, and here the arms. Fingers and toes, size of the head, the growth just right for the stated number of weeks. Holding hands, smiling with confidence, Maggie and I alternately glanced at each other and at the screen. The beam was pointed at the heart. We watched a rhythmic series of wave forms, little pointed bumps, stream across the screen. Some waves looked bigger than others. That was unfamiliar. I didn't remember that from the other ultrasounds I had seen.

In the darkened room, watching the grey and white forms scroll across the screen, a fleeting moment had departed from the script.

Foreboding crept up on me. I scanned my memories of previous ultrasounds, trying to reassure myself that the images on the screen were normal.

But something was wrong.

My heart paused, afraid, behind my ribs. Time stood still. A sudden tight seal held the dark room adrift from the ordinary passage of life. I felt a gripping in my chest as the world seemed to empty of everything but the question at hand. A confused mixture of déjà vu and half-remembered images blended to produce uncertainty, and fear.

I struggled to voice my unease: 'Uh ... umm... Is... Excuse me? Is that ... normal? It looks a bit ... Is that wave a bit ... small?'

The sonographer, glancing my way, paused to clarify the question, as I pointed at the screen. She tilted her head and waited for me to speak. Nervous, I rephrased the question in my mind, before wondering aloud, 'Isn't the, is the, the amplitude of that heart signal ... a bit low?

'No,' the woman paused, 'it's all okay'. Adjusting her hands slightly. 'I think it's just the angle of the transducer.' She manipulated the probe for another look. 'You can see there's a normal heartbeat there. We had a nice four-chamber view just before.'

The experienced sonographer was unruffled. My choking feeling faded. Her murmured reassurance was effective. My alarm, I reminded myself, was based on very limited experience. The moment passed. Restart the clock—unfreeze the time, we're back at our breeding best! My unease grew faint in a handful of seconds. Breath returned and smiling resumed.

That one moment, suffused with destiny, sank back to join countless others in the file of obscured memories. Most of those memories will never be retrieved. That one moment is with me now, at my desk. It forces its way back. What if I'd acted then and there to demand a closer look or a second opinion? What if I'd been decisive and trusted my gut feeling? What if I had declined to be reassured?

If I had more experience with ultrasound, could I have known what was in store? Could we have been better prepared?

That frozen moment belongs in a cluster of dysphoric flash-backs; a set of destructive memories. They are labelled by their type: THE WHAT IFs.

2

IT'S A BOY

*Things which matter most must never be at the mercy
of things which matter least.*

— Goethe

Embarrassing stories about President Bill Clinton flooded
the media for months on end, but in February 1999 he was
acquitted by the Senate in his impeachment trial. That same
month, Eminem released his first major album, *The Slim Shady
LP*. By March, Roberto Benigni and Gwyneth Paltrow were
preparing to accept the Academy Awards for Best Actor and Best
Actress, for their roles in *Life is Beautiful* and *Shakespeare in Love*,
respectively.

Meanwhile in Australia, Maggie Frawley went through the
nesting process one more time, for an event of much greater
importance in our lives. The second day of March would see the
birth of our fourth and youngest child, Malachy Declan Mandela
Frawley. Feeling quite certain this would end our breeding season,
we couldn't resist slipping in a tip of the hat to Nelson Mandela, the
great freedom fighter of our lifetime.

Myriad challenges no doubt beset our young family every day
through that period, but none of them weighed on us unduly. The
future was unquestionably ours to grasp, and with four young
children in tow (very shortly) we had neither the time nor the
inclination to doubt our readiness for the grand adventure ahead.

They were peaceful days, but there was a freight train heading our way, the rushing fury and power of its approach inexplicably silent. Any gods watching must have stared through the cracks between their spectral fingers, dismayed at our blissful lack of anticipation.

The labour to deliver Malachy, undertaken at our local district hospital, was strenuous but uneventful. Maggie had hoped for that easy brisk delivery we'd had friends speak of, but not yet experienced in three attempts. Subsequent children were supposed to find their way into the world more easily than their elders, but not for us. Again, with number four, Maggie laboured throughout the night, with support from me and one of her close friends, Jenny. Malachy was delivered safely on the morning of 2nd March, with the attendance of experienced midwives and a local GP, who was a friend from the nearby town of Berry. The night's efforts left us all in a haze of exhaustion and excitement. After an initial check-over with doctor and midwife, Maggie and Malachy were transferred to the maternity ward of Nowra Community Hospital.

Not contemplating rest, nor hearing the rumble of the figurative freight train, I picked up the children from home where their cousin Lucy had babysat the long productive night. Bundled into the car, off to meet their new brother, were Imogen, in her Size 5 school uniform, three-and-a-half-year-old Seamus and Niamh, still herself a baby at 20 months. We all leapt out for an early morning hospital visit and our first photo opportunity with Malachy.

Niamh was ever so nervous as she climbed up into the low floral armchair, positioning herself to allow the brand-new bundle of brother to be balanced across her lap. Captured on film, her look is nonplussed. The strange living doll is warm and squirmy as Niamh lets her arms flop, unable to master nursing. In that first photo, Seamus has craned into view fascinated, delighted, his deeply tanned arms looping forward, where his index finger pokes delicately into the grasping palm of his newly minted playmate. Imogen, older and more competent, compliantly eager to please as she had always been, mastered the cradling task after a brief hesitation. This boy was only a curiosity for now, but in time she would cradle, carry, comfort, capture and cajole him at every opportunity. The warm sleeping collection of swaddling left Imogen beaming at the camera, a euphoric wave of pleasure sweeping her along involuntarily. Love swept us all up in its blind intoxication.

Maggie went off to sleep while I went home, also planning to sleep. But adrenaline dictated that instead of sleep, I ring everyone I could think of to gloat about the safe arrival of our tallest baby, rivalling in beauty the earlier masterpieces. The thrill and satisfaction of completing our long-planned family buzzed through my weary brain as I finally succumbed, settling into a deep slumber.

Minutes later I woke to the urgent imperative of our home telephone.

While I'd been splashing our ecstatic news far and wide, Maggie fell into a recovery slumber. Malachy's crib was out at the nurses' station, ensuring peace and quiet for the new mum. It wasn't going so well for Malachy. Sister Helen had noted a dusky colour to the Frawley infant. A whiff of oxygen did little to improve his hue, and the oxygen level measured in his tiny fingertips registered an unexpectedly low score. While I was at home blithely crossing off one sibling then another from my list of calls, a drama was unfolding. Two doctors, an anaesthetist, Rob, and a paediatrician, Toby, had been summoned, drips inserted, and a set of X-rays ordered.

All the while Maggie slept.

Nothing the professionals did seemed to improve the appearance of this baby who had at first seemed a picture of perfection. In the unseen workings of newborn physiology, the oxygen that baby Malachy breathed had triggered a normal chain of events, transforming his circulation from that of a foetus to that of a neonate. While cocooned in Maggie's womb her lungs had given Malachy all the oxygen he needed, passing oxygen through the placenta with no need for the baby to breathe. Once he was delivered his own lungs and circulation would need to take over.

This brings us to the crux of the great 'What if'. That uncomfortable moment in the ultrasound suite had an explanation.

Malachy's heart had no valve opening to the lungs, hence no normal route to pump blood through the life-giving bellows. To get oxygen, Malachy relied instead on blood flow through the *ductus arteriosus*, a remnant of his foetal circulation. As the chemistry of newborn life worked its transforming magic minute by minute, Malachy's *ductus arteriosus* closed. This is normal. In a normal baby this closure makes the transition to healthy circulation complete, allowing the right ventricle of the heart to pump blood straight into the lung circulation. As Malachy's altered anatomy offered no other route into the lungs, an open *ductus arteriosus* was essential to his survival—its closure meant that Malachy's only way to oxygenate his body had disappeared.

With a violent hissing of brakes and steam billowing wildly as it crashed into the safety bollards, that freight train had arrived. If we had known what was coming, Malachy would not have been delivered in our small rural hospital, but in Sydney, straight into the waiting hands of intensive care experts. No delays and no surprises.

In my memory, the ringing of the phone that morning has taken on the screeching quality of an alarm. Shocked and stammering, I recognised the voice of the paediatrician on the line. 'Dom, it's Toby here. I've been called to look at your baby who the nursing staff observed to be cyanosed. He has central cyanosis, and his X-ray shows an enlarged heart. I think your baby has cyanotic heart disease, quite possibly Tetralogy of Fallot.[1]

Minutes later, after a stricken car trip to the hospital, it fell to me to bring this news to Maggie. I tapped lightly and entered the peaceful shelter of the room. Maggie stirred, turning her face towards me, serenity and weariness in equal measure. 'Malachy is

---

1   Tetralogy of Fallot is the most common form of cyanotic congenital heart disease. The term 'tetralogy' refers to the presence of a combination of four different heart defects. The effect of the four defects is to produce low oxygenation, breathing distress, cyanosis of the skin and a 'boot-shaped' heart on Xray. Malachy had all those signs, but not the underlying Tetralogy.

at the nurse's station,' she murmured as she reached an arm out for an embrace. Warm as toast in her dream-like state, as Maggie touched my shoulder, she joined me at a point of no return.

'I know, darling, he's at the nurses' station, but he's not so well. There's something wrong. It looks like Malachy has a heart problem. Toby and Rob are both out there looking after him. They've called the helicopter. They have to send him to Sydney.'

The inner white noise of collision drowned everything.

The photos we had taken earlier that morning now carry the emotional weight of last capture—the last moments of normal life, a life which was soon to be divided into eras. As nature closed Malachy's *ductus arteriosus*, our life split in two.

Depicted are the last moments of 'Before'. Everything else is 'After'.

That day became a blur as events marched forward. I recall a flurry of discussion about the wind conditions and whether or not Maggie could join Malachy in the Care Flight helicopter to Sydney. I watched on helplessly as Maggie disappeared into the cramped cabin of the chopper, followed by Malachy, his ambulance trolley bearing him in the clear plastic shell of an emergency crib. The care of the other children needed sorting, with their cousin Lucy stepping in while I borrowed her car and drove alone through the dark, following the chopper.

The destination was Sydney Children's Hospital, where Malachy had all manner of drains and tubes pushed into his tiny body and was tested and retested to make a diagnosis. Maggie and I went through one detailed discussion after another and watched a range of staff dart in with various interventions to keep Malachy stable. We stared for hours at our unconscious baby, listened to the doctors and nurses, and stared at the walls of interview rooms.

3

INTENSE BEGINNINGS

If you are going through hell, keep going.

— Winston Churchill

On 3rd March I woke at first light. The struts of a fold-out bed had made their presence felt through the night. I creaked and strained my way into consciousness and breathed in the stale hospital air of Maggie's room at the Royal Hospital for Women. The main bed was empty. The emerging light of morning drew me to the window. I lurched suddenly. I choked, then sobbed. My body convulsed in waves as I realised where I was. I doubled over again as I realised why. Like a mute animal I leaked salt water from nose and eyes as stifled howls filled my chest. My tears would not stop, my eyes would not focus.

This must be what unbearable pain is like. Perhaps it's universal? Such suffering is lonely. The world came down to this one point in which I could not make sense of my altered state.

Is this my life now?

I sensed a presence. Turning to my right Maggie was standing still, fragile, her eyes reddened, watching with a veneer of calm.

'I wondered if you would have the same reaction as me,' she said gently.

Maggie had let me sleep, reasoning that I would need the rest after the distress of the preceding day. This was a pattern of caring that would sustain me in the trials ahead. I wanted, in turn, to be that same kind of rock for her.

By rights Malachy could have been called a 'blue baby', the traditional term for a baby whose heart could not deliver enough oxygen to his body. Oxygen turns blood pink. As it is used up, the blood and hence the baby, turns blue.

The lack of oxygen puts a blue baby at high risk of complications. Every cell in Malachy's body was short of oxygen. His gut became susceptible to gangrene and infections. His liver strained to cope, leading to jaundice. While unconscious, the effects on his brain could not be known. Unable to mount a strong cough, his lungs clogged with secretions.

After four days Malachy wasn't straight blue, but rather red, yellow and blue. His body, wracked with pain and arched in distress, was like a national flag for sick babies; a brightly contrasted line demarcating his red, infected abdomen from his yellow, jaundiced chest, while the tips of everything stayed obstinately blue.

Even after many years, the feel and smell, the air of disaster, still seem within touching distance. I can close my eyes and absorb once more the tension of not knowing, the powerlessness and the callous spotlessness of intensive care, with its soundtrack of beeps, blips and alarms. Still in my bones is the huddled gloom of the parents in the dreaded morning lockout while the doctors do their ward round. Each morning, hospital rules saw family members ejected from the Intensive Care Unit, to allow the doctors and nurses to speak freely about their critically sick patients. We were all forced out into a tiny anteroom with no facilities but a cramped row of chairs lining the walls.

I hope this dreaded cupboard off the main corridor at Sydney Children's Hospital has changed in the years since, but in 1999 while the daily ward round was in progress, eight to 12 sleep-deprived, desperately worried parents had to share half a dozen chairs in a windowless corral, exchanging horror stories about their children while nursing their own fears behind a brave exterior.

It was often quite testing as the morning drew on and people's frustrations and worries about their children boiled over, without any capacity to seek redress.

Combing back through the memory of those early months of Malachy's life there is an image that forces itself forward, that crystallises what it felt like to be that parent, watching your beloved child struggle and suffer. Even now I shudder at the image I carry of my parched, toxic baby wracked by infection, fever, pain and dehydration. An organism barely conscious recognising only an instinct to live on.

Malachy's headline problem was his malformed heart. This vulnerable organ was responsible for delivery of oxygen to every other cell in his body. Nature's design would have us cry our way through our newborn period, plump and pink, our blood fully saturated with life-bringing oxygen to drop off at each needy organ in turn. When that doesn't work, those organs have to make do. If there is almost normal oxygen, your circulation works a bit harder, and you get by. With not quite enough, the struggle is more obvious, the system strains, the risks climb. Once you're clearly under-supplied, there is trouble, as we would discover.

Somewhere in the barrage of days that ushered Malachy into the world, as X-ray mounted on blood test and line after tube after drain were inserted and removed, Malachy developed a fever. Samples were taken to look for a culprit bacteria, as antibiotics were added on presumption of the likely organism, while he grew sicker. As the results arrived to advise a change was needed, that we won't win with these drugs, the tipping point was reached. His bowel, starved of oxygen and fighting off gangrene had started to die by degrees, signalled by a deepening red colour that lit the entire lower half of his body, stretching the skin shiny, brightly inflamed. Simultaneously the toxicity enveloped other functions as the fever rose, the struggling heart raced, and a deep yellow jaundice coloured his upper chest and back. Onto this red and yellow banner of human tissue came the gently probing hands of the surgical registrar. The moment froze in time. Malachy arched in pain as the trained fingers sounded out the festering mess within. His mouth fell open, part agony, part air hunger, dry tongue and lips mutely crying for help.

This image lives on.

Enmeshed as I was in this battle for survival, I knew this life to be in the balance and that the path ahead would demand surgical intervention.

When the surgical verdict came down it carried the ominous name 'necrotising enterocolitis'[2]. As the seriousness of Malachy's condition was explained the surgeon revealed the consensus view was that our boy was so unstable, so fragile, that the hospital would not risk transferring him down the corridor to the operating theatres. He was instead to be cut open right there in ICU. In the surgeon's words, 'If we don't operate, he will die of this infection'.

So it passed that 'Mac', as he would be known, had his first operation when he was four days old. Not on his heart, but rather to remove a stretch of gangrenous bowel, a casualty of his hapless circulation.

On the day of Mac's surgery, he became the reason all parents were herded out for prolonged exclusion from the Intensive Care Unit, which was now a sterile operating theatre. Long after the morning ward round was completed, our baby was still lying open on the operating table as the surgeons wrestled with diseased tissue to reclose the wounds they had inflicted. As tense as it may have been for all those parents, they did not force their pain on us. Perhaps it was our equivalent of battlefield solidarity—for we all found ourselves in this mess together. That day it was our turn to be that hapless family about which people can reflect, 'No matter

---

2 Necrotising enterocolitis (NEC) is a devastating disease that affects mostly the intestine of sick babies, especially where there is a low oxygen level. The wall of the intestine is infected by bacteria, which can destroy the tissues, resulting in perforation of the bowel wall and life-threatening sepsis.

how bad it gets, in here you can always find someone whose child is worse off than yours'.

By the time the doors were opened, the news for us was that Malachy had lost a segment of bowel and still had extensive infection to combat. Malachy's bowel had been diverted to a 'stoma', an opening through the wall of his abdomen, where the bowel fed out through his skin into a colostomy bag.

Nonetheless, yes, he was alive.

4

SHUNTED

Eye contact: how souls catch fire.

— Yahia Lababidi

Day five dawned, and it wouldn't be accurate to say Malachy's recovery was uncomplicated. Certainly, the spreading gangrene of his bowel was arrested and the antibiotics were working their scientific magic, bringing the infection under control. Mac's vital signs were settling into a rhythm, but our baby still had blood tests and X-rays every day. Multiple tubes ran to and from his body, meeting his needs for breathing, treatment, nutrition, monitoring and excretion. He still had regular bouts of suction in which the nursing staff fed long plastic tubes down into his airways to suck out the messy secretions he was unable to cough up. He still had countless measures of every sign of life, every millilitre of urine, every dose of a plethora of drugs, every drop of fluid balance issued carefully and documented in detail.

All that careful watching was part of nursing him to recovery from his unplanned emergency operation. That procedure was marked on his body by wide rubbery-looking dressings that hid the incision line from one side of his abdomen to the other and by the colostomy bag, sealed to his skin to catch the produce from his shortened bowel. Malachy was yet to face his planned operation.

Feeding in through a large vein in Malachy's groin was what is known as a femoral central venous line. This is a specialised type of 'drip', the more familiar type of needle often placed somewhere in an arm vein to feed a patient fluid and drugs. A femoral line is able to remain in place much longer than ordinary drips, is wide enough to have more than one 'lumen', or channel, and is fed into the largest vein in the body, the inferior vena cava, or IVC. The IVC is big enough to allow noxious chemicals to be fed into the bloodstream without as much risk as usual of corroding the vessel. Malachy's tiny femoral vein was just large enough to accommodate the insertion of the femoral line.

One of the drugs being fed in through Malachy's groin was Prostaglandin. This wonder drug, fairly recently developed, was keeping Malachy alive by holding open his *ductus arteriosus*. Without this drug, the ductus would close, plunging Malachy back into the type of crisis we had witnessed on day one at our local hospital. As days passed the risk increased that nature would override the effect of the Prostaglandin, so it became imperative to avoid undue delay of an operation for his heart.

Gary Sholler, the cardiologist, and the cardiac surgeon, Graham Nunn, advised us that Mac needed a procedure to create an artificial blood vessel or 'shunt' to divert blood from his body into his lung circulation. On its return to the heart from the lungs, this blood would then mix with the blood returning from the body, to make partially oxygenated blood, to send back out around the body. The doctors emphasised this would not be perfect as normal hearts have two pumping chambers, or ventricles, for a reason. But Malachy's anatomy was so malformed that functional, not perfect, was the goal.

All the while Malachy was kept sedated, buried in his struggle for survival with painkillers and sedatives added to the more technical aspects of his treatment. He couldn't be detached from the life-preserving apparatus surrounding him so remained impossible to hold or hug. His eyes remained steadfastly closed.

A narrow window of time beckoned. Malachy needed to be adequately recovered from his bowel surgery to handle having his chest cut open, but he couldn't wait too long because his *ductus arteriosus* would close, spelling disaster.

Our other children came and went, in the temporary care of rallied family and friends. Visitors came and went too, each contributing something special of their own to a wave of goodwill sweeping us along. The daily rhythm of tests and discussions, ward-round lockouts, and arrivals and departures of yet more sick babies and distraught parents rolled on. The ambience of neon lighting was relentless, as day was hardly distinguished from night. The to and fro along barren hallways to meet our needs for sleep or sustenance, or to express breast milk, then back to care for our stricken baby, seemed endless.

Through all of this, something started to niggle at Maggie and me. After more than a week, Malachy had never voluntarily opened his eyes. Nurses had prised open his eyelids to force the glare of torchlight through. Presumably, this was to confirm the presence of brain function. There had been no visual bonding; no loving stares between parent and child were given or received. A maze of tubes and cords made cuddles a no-go, leaving stroking small available patches of skin about as good as it got. What meaning we attach to our eyes! Can you really pour love into a child through this bejewelled portal? It dragged on; our baby couldn't see us at all, and we had no window to his soul.

One morning early, a gift lay on the table at the base of Malachy's crib. One of those special people, able to bring a light heart to a hard place, had nursed our boy through the neon harshness of another night. A pile of Polaroid photos taken through the night bore the title: *What Does Malachy Do When His Parents Are Asleep?*

We paged through a series of stop-motion photos with some soft toys assembling on Malachy's bed, and a Pelican daring to venture closer, closer, to the head of the human. The pelican appears to whisper in Mac's ear. What was said will remain between the two of them but what we saw on the final page was unmistakable. A strip of deep blue-black colour had opened up below the brow, as the toy pelican leaned in for a response. There seemed no doubt that here in truth was an open eye, for the first time, witnessed by Mr Pelican.

The next day, with Malachy around ten days old, the surgeon got the green light to proceed with the shunting operation, opening a wound running between two of Malachy's ribs, wrapping around the left-hand side of his back. With Mac's ribs held open by his surgical assistants, Graham successfully manipulated the minute vessels to achieve the desired outcome, ensuring safe blood flow into Malachy's lungs. The procedure he performed was the installation of a Blalock-Taussig shunt. This was an operation conceived in 1943 and given some degree of fame as a focal point in the 2004 movie *Something the Lord Made*. The movie depicts the development of the shunting procedure through the bravery and genius of three people in the US: a laboratory technician named Vivien Thomas, with the surgeon Alfred Blalock and cardiologist Helen Taussig. Their reach into the future had that day saved Malachy's life.

After such an arduous and complex period of suspense, each day was happier than the one before as Malachy first pulled through the operation, then was progressively relieved of one tube or catheter after another. Gradually he needed fewer drugs and less monitoring. As the treatment eased off, the sedation lightened.

When he was two weeks old, Malachy opened his eyes and stared at his parents, obviously unaware of the profound effect this novel action had on them. His eyes had the expected deep, baby blue colour, which would in time be replaced by the brown he inherited from me.

On day 15, with Malachy more alert, and with one less line attached to his tiny body, Maggie was allowed a moment she had been craving. A chair was positioned next to the crib, and the drip stands all moved beside the chair. Maggie was guided to the chair. The plastic tubing was freed of tangles and a pillow placed on her lap. Onto that pillow Malachy was placed. There, mother and son would enjoy their first embrace since the chain of disaster was set in motion. We have a photo of that moment when Mac could first receive a physical demonstration of love, of something other than a medical or surgical salvage procedure. Maggie is looking upward into the camera with an uncertain air born of the preceding trauma, mixed with relief. The blue of her eyes is striking next to the lingering rings of redness. Layers of meaning seem to stare through the camera as, cradled afloat on a pillow is a tiny, blue-pink bundle, string-like tubes trailing off towards the adjacent drip stand. I felt overwhelmed with tenderness for both of them, the woman who had steadfastly endured every drama, all the while unable to hold or caress her featherweight child, and the boy who, in his battle, had carved himself so deeply into my psyche.

By the time Malachy was laid out on his mother's lap, Maggie and I felt as though we'd been through a lifetime of sombre discussions, of sleepless nights, of consoling distressed relatives and bolstering each other. Malachy's life had hung by a thread from hour to hour, day to day, and we had grown accustomed to the intensity of watching for every movement, every change, any sign that the balance had tipped either for or against this tiny suffering creature.

The bond of love for a child is so rarely tested to this degree. Under this kind of duress you are forced to realise with great clarity just how much you love them. It created a profound distillation of the essence of parental love; That a human being I hardly knew, who had never spoken a word to me, could move me so powerfully. One friend of mine suggested that babies like Malachy, or threats to the life of any one of your children, 'Make you want to hug them harder'.

Basking in the joy of being able to cradle and nurture our boy and to finally share a mutual gaze, we made little of various complications. Among these was some minor damage to Malachy's femoral artery, the major vessel supplying blood to his right leg.

It was also found that the femoral line, so essential to delivering treatment to the infant, having fitted so snugly in the blood vessel, had caused a clot to form, completely blocking the major vein to the heart, the inferior vena cava.

This blockage would prove to be another 'What if?' as events unfolded.

5

GREY WORLD

You can't run away from trouble.
There ain't no place that far.

— Uncle Remus

Long hours and interminable days were played out in mere survival mode by us and many others in ICU. Maggie and I had to look deep into each other's eyes and confirm that we would survive regardless of the outcome; that we could handle whatever happened. We developed a code between us, an understanding that our future could not be ruined beyond redemption by Malachy's death or disability. There was a current of something carrying us along, a resilience, a grim persistence of hope in the face of having no good straws to clutch. This we came to know as our 'god of good outcomes'—a concept, or being, we would be grateful to more than once.

Maggie's challenge in dealing with Malachy was compounded by her own postnatal condition. She wrestled with the ordeal of maintaining breast milk, having to express and gather her milk in small plastic jars for a baby unable to suckle. The jars were stored in a dedicated fridge in the maternity ward in the adjoining Women's Hospital, there being no beds for recovery from childbirth in a children's hospital. It was up to us to carry the milk across to the ICU, ensuring it remained suitably well preserved. Malachy would, in turn, have Maggie's milk warmed, then syringed into his mouth by a nurse. Maggie was also enduring the whole upheaval of recovering from a birth made harder by finding the midwives missing in action, seemingly terrified of dealing with a grief-stricken parent. I can understand. Many people would find it easier nursing happy mothers with well babies through to their discharge home rather than the constantly tearful, preoccupied woman in the end room.

Maggie's wing at the Royal Women's was linked to Sydney Children's by long barren corridors. At one end Maggie wrestled with milk supply and her own recovery, while at the other, Malachy survived septic infection, cardiac arrest, bowel surgery, numerous visitors, two Catholic sacraments and who remembers what more.

Somewhere around this time, our red-eyed reverie was interrupted with a venture to a local café. A small group of our Nowra friends had made the three-hour trip to Randwick to lend their support. Stepping outside gave us our first taste of fresh air since the birth. With our friends we trudged around the corner from the hospital and found a place with an outdoor table and a little shade where we sat down and traded our stories of disaster babies. Each of our friends had had babies who needed intensive care, so life and death was the topic of our musings. Such sadness I had never desired to know.

The conversation turned to coping. 'How do you cope?' is a perennial favourite question offered to newborn disaster parents. The theory was quietly advanced that the correct answer to that chestnut is, 'I didn't know I had a choice'. Daring to see a road ahead, the group then embarked tentatively onto the troubled waters of black humour—hospital version. That's where you joke about the foibles of nurses, the pretensions of doctors, and the near misses survived. The silly comment someone made during your son's resuscitation suddenly seems amusing more than offensive. We emitted brief chuckles through the veils heavy around our hearts.

Undetected, something snuck its way through the gloom, like a good fairy deftly tickling inside my chest. A dam burst, and the gentle reflective ironies gave way to laughter. Primal laughter. A seemingly long-forgotten brightness was complemented by sunshine breaking through the heavy skies, landing on our table. We laughed until the tears rolled down our faces, well beyond just remembering what it felt like to laugh, the pain in my sides didn't stop me at all. Joy had asserted itself. Colour lived on in this grey-shaded world.

6

CATHETER

You know, 97 percent of the time, if you come into a hospital, everything goes well. But three percent of the time, we have major complications.

— Atul Gawande

Malachy first made it home to Nowra on a bright autumn day, nearly four weeks old. I made a rushed last-minute purchase of an esky. With all the focus on our baby we had overlooked the precious collection of expressed breast milk Maggie had been amassing while her child was labelled, **NIL BY MOUTH**. It was a comforting time, being welcomed home into the support of our local community, and then re-establishing a domestic rhythm. Childhood heart disease is often not a one-off episode of treatment. This is unlike, for example, many cancers, where the life and death struggle is fearsome for a stretch of time, and the battle either won or lost. Congenital heart disease never goes away. Malachy's medical care had bursts of intensity and high-risk procedures, interspersed with expectant lulls. Get sick, get fixed, watch and wait. Repeat unpredictably.

Our settled period was uninterrupted for a month. When Malachy was two months old we signed him in for another procedure, to find out exactly what his anatomy was, and whether it needed fixing. The plan was to inject contrast dye into his circulation, lighting up the structure of the heart in stark relief on

X-ray images. The 'cardiac catheter' is a highly specialised medical shadow theatre, amazing for an outsider to watch, but considered routine within the intense world of paediatric cardiology.

Living through the intermittent disaster of rearing an infant with heart disease, I found that operations could be strangely soothing. While Malachy was hidden away on an operating table there was some time to focus, all petty concerns were erased, and my only company was often Maggie, or those closest to Maggie and me. The waiting time was spent sharing profound concern for Mac's welfare.

During surgery we felt the consolation that Malachy was in good hands. A gathering of highly trained experts were all intently working on our precious child, hidden from view. All we had to do was wait. In due course we learnt to cover our apprehension by seeking out a meal, chewing carefully, tasting slowly, safe in the knowledge that we were free for at least the length of time the doctors had predicted. The elephant in the room could sit ignored for an interlude.

Paediatric hospital resources were not evenly spread in Sydney.

We learnt that the doctors were starting to prefer performing heart surgery at Westmead rather than Randwick. The Westmead hospital was supported by the lion's share of funding. From a parent's perspective both hospitals had their merits.

I liked Randwick, having worked there in the early nineties. At Randwick it was much easier to get away from the confines of the hospital, with access to a variety of nearby parks and gardens and a myriad of dining options to pass the time. If you could escape from the hospital for long enough you could almost pretend it was 'business as usual'.

At Westmead, we parents were pretty much trapped inside the hospital. There were just two food outlets: the tasty one or the budget one. I found it harder to get a sense of distance from our worries. Having said that, the designers and planners had worked hard to make the new children's hospital as pleasant as possible. In Mac's stays there I found the walls had been scattered liberally with the works of famous artists. Many of their pieces were tactile and child-friendly and were interspersed with naive works by schoolchildren or hospital patients. Outside Intensive Care, for example, was a brilliant John Olsen, neighbouring enthusiastic imitations from the children of Sydney. It helped brighten up the halls of medical misery. In some of our worrying times the gallery effect buoyed me by displaying community concern for the suffering of children.

Hidden around the hospital are also some design follies and secret nooks such as a fountain and pergola, some play equipment you can play a tune on, and life-size sculptures of workers abseiling from the wave-like rooftop of the main building. I recall once having the sense I was lost in a design masterpiece as I turned down a vaulted corridor with bold overlapping ceiling structures, slanting walls and elegant pylons stretching skyward behind an expanse of plated glass.

Walking those designer halls is the kind of thing Maggie and I were doing that day in May.

The planned cardiac catheter was a minor, day procedure so we didn't have to mark too much time. We drifted towards the main entrance, watching the busy passing mix of patients, parents and health professionals. We ordered a coffee from a stall as we shared the inescapable tension of the day and, with our default set to 'optimism', settled in to wait.

Lost in the bustle, distractedly surveying the child-friendly design, our reverie was interrupted by an insistent male voice moving rapidly around the foyer area: 'The Frawleys. Are the Frawleys here? Dom and Maggie Frawley? Are you the Frawleys?'

Here comes gravity ... WHACK. That's us he's after. He looks flustered. He's out of breath.

'Yes, we're the Frawleys. What's going on? We're not expecting you yet... Sure, we'll follow you'... etc. While chasing the nurse back through the corridors to find the catheter lab we were briefed that something had gone wrong, the cardiologist needed to talk to us, urgently. In a strange haze I also recall making hurried small talk with the nurse as we rushed our way to the theatre. My dim recollection is of being bemused, in the midst of disaster, to find myself hearing that the nurse was once married to my distant cousin. From his standpoint, any small talk was better than having to tell us what we would soon discover. Turning the last corner, Dr Sholler waited in surgical scrubs, beaded sweat on his flushed face below the rim of a paper hat.

Carefully, but speedily, Gary Sholler told us that Malachy had had a cardiac arrest during the procedure, which is bad, but been successfully resuscitated, which is good. Dr Sholler hadn't been able to get the information he needed yet, which is bad, but thought useful knowledge was attainable by pressing ahead, despite the dangers, which is good. He needed our consent to proceed. We gave consent—what choice did we have?

A simple planning procedure had become a harrowing setback. Mac left the catheter lab unconscious on a trolley, bound once more for Intensive Care, in a tiny skullcap of white padding to preserve heat en route. The doctor advised us he had remained stable after our doorstop interview, but nonetheless needed closer monitoring. We followed the trolley and monitors to the ICU, where verbal notes were passed on, observations relayed, and history recollected for a new group of expert carers. As the professional banter progressed there was a sudden beeping and a change to the cadence of Mac's monitors, a noticeable stiffening of spines all round, then some yelling, 'He's arrested!', and a flurry of chest pummelling and airway manipulations.

Maggie and I were three metres away, watching the disaster unfold, knowing not to plunge in and risk cluttering up the workspace or slowing the life-saving treatment. There we were, embracing each other in stunned silence, tears falling from our faces in hopeless protest, when the exclamation cut across our senses: 'They're crying—get the social worker'.

It showed the best and worst of how a big hospital system makes people react. Humanity can become a problem. Our normal, healthy tears apparently needed urgent fixing by a professional.

We possibly needed a social worker. Malachy certainly needed intensive care.

There truly is a specialist for every human need.

7

A HOLE AND A HIERARCHY

It is the little things that pierce and burn and prick for years to come.

— Algernon Blackwood

The stark lights of the paediatric Intensive Care illuminated another forlorn scene in our boy's hectic, short two months of life. Splinted to ensure its movement wouldn't dislodge a dripline, Malachy's right arm stretched toward us. Two towers of medical delivery devices rose at the bedhead, one on either side. Lights flashed intermittently, numbers lit up on the face of each device, and high-pitched sounds alerted the staff to any hiccups in function. Further monitors recorded and displayed each beat of Mac's heart, the ups and downs of his breath, his blood pressure, his pulse, his oxygen levels. The devices fed in fluids and drugs to take external control of umpteen bodily functions once again.

Following Malachy's complicated catheter study and the cardiac arrest, it was established that his current problem was due to changes occurring inside his heart. The success of his earlier shunt procedure depended on being able to mix the blood returning to his heart from both body and lungs in a single upper chamber, or atrium, of the heart. A normal heart has two atria, left and right, separated by a wall, or septum. In order to mix the returning blood, Malachy needed a hole through the septum. Fortunately, he did have a hole there, through a window known as the *foramen ovale*.

34

This natural hole normally closes in the first few days of life, but sometimes persists for six months or more. At two months, Malachy would be better off if his *foramen ovale* stayed open, but this closure was happening now, and quickly. As it shrank, the passage of blood back from Malachy's body was being choked off, making life precarious. While a hole in the heart is something many people know is dangerous, Malachy's specific problem meant that his heart not only needed a hole, it needed a bigger hole.

Dr Sholler addressed this problem by inviting the surgeon to undertake another operation. This time not a mere shunt, but open-heart surgery. To open up the required channel between Malachy's atria, Dr Nunn operated to remove the whole atrial septum, in a procedure called 'atrial septectomy'. This involved sawing through the front of the chest and opening up Malachy's sternum, producing the 'zipper' scar so emblematic of children with major heart defects.

Surgery of this scale required intensive post-operative care and recovery which carried with it enormous risks. Malachy would need to steady a bit before being well enough to proceed. With risks come complications. We'd already had complications aplenty.

The complex drama of those days was not limited to Malachy. We had other children, and Maggie had given birth just two months ago. She maintained a heartfelt determination to breastfeed Malachy, reasoning that he needed the nutritional and immune benefits of colostrum and breast milk, possibly more than any normal child. This required session after session of working away on breast pumps to gather the necessary milk, which we would then rely on the nursing staff to administer to Malachy. In the course of our stay Maggie, in her exhaustion, had gone to have a sleep in the parents' room, returning to find to her distress one of the nurses feeding Malachy formula milk. Maggie burst into tears as the nurse explained she was trying to allow her some rest. After two months of fighting to maintain her supply of milk and provide Malachy with her own supply of nutrient, carefully delaying his exposure to cow's milk, Maggie was thwarted by an act of misplaced kindness. It was just the kind of unintended consequence that beleaguers hospital systems. A small indignity caused by assumption or failure of communication. Just the kind of thing that keeps parents on edge.

Each little frustration was understandable or excusable in itself, but the net effect of one after another, after another, was taking its toll. Especially when so much else was out of control.

With an ache, I recall the blockage of Malachy's vena cava, which had seemed of little account in the drama of his first month of life. Dr Sholler's catheter procedure had confirmed the blockage and the absence of any clearing of the clot, which now permanently closed off the vessel. This precluded the ability to pass a central line in through Malachy's groin: the preferred site of entry for the necessary drugs.

A central line was deemed important, so the anaesthetists and intensive care doctors had set to work on Malachy, seeking to pass a line in through his neck instead, through the jugular vein. Maggie and I waited in the corridor while Malachy was sedated and draped and the bed tilted feet up, to help send a rush of blood to enlarge the targeted veins. His head flushed, engorged with blood as the doctor passed a large needle into the base of his neck, and failed to place it correctly. Our consent was sought and given to continue. With blood staining his gloves and Malachy's skin, the doctor tried and failed again, while we waited, powerless to help or protect. Then the procedure failed again.

We had reached one excusable setback too many.

Maggie exploded: 'You have to stop! You clearly can't do what you're trying to do. He's my son. You're going to kill him if you don't back off.'

People rushed to placate, defend and excuse. Someone crossed a line into condescension. It seemed pride was at stake. It seems incredible that anyone working in that critical environment could ever forget that to a parent whose child's life is at stake, professional defensiveness is like a red rag to a bull. So it proved.

Led by Maggie we demanded the team rethink their strategy and find someone who could successfully install the needed line. There were some similar irritations as the day proceeded, creating something of a stand-off between us and the professionals, until we were approached for a meeting with a senior doctor.

A sheepish, humble manner suggested the doctor was in peacemaker mode. His open body language, designed to reduce feelings of threat, was taken straight from my first year Behavioural Sciences tutorials at Sydney University. Maggie had studied similar methods in her teacher training. Textbook, too, was his opening.

'Mrs Frawley, you seem to be angry'.

'Of course, I'm angry! My child is sick and I'm being shut out of the room while you do one thing after another to him.'

'So, what is it that you're angry about?'

'I just told you what I'm angry about. Why won't you listen?'

'I am listening to you. I know you're worr—'

'You're not listening. You've obviously been sent to calm me down, but that's not the point. The point is you're messing up the care of our child. You can't fix Malachy by trying to calm me down.'

The procedure ended up being abandoned. Instead of a central line, Malachy received two additional, smaller, peripheral venous drips.

Malachy's heart continued to struggle and by the next day, recurrent dips in blood pressure and strain on his heart indicated an urgent need to press on with the surgical repair. After careful discussions with Dr Sholler, and with Dr Winlaw from the surgical team, we couldn't avoid the conclusion that the risk of waiting outstripped the hazards of open-heart surgery. The septectomy was arranged with our consent, and Malachy was trolleyed off to the operating theatres. Maggie and I had no choice but to explore the hospital once more—this operation would take several hours.

The atrial septum was removed successfully, with the operation running smoothly by Dr Nunn's account. The obstructing tissue was removed, but Malachy had suffered a heart attack somewhere in the preceding days, damaging part of his heart muscle. He returned to ICU with still more tubing attached to his body, now including drains implanted into his chest cavity and pacemaker leads to his heart. His sternum had been sawn open then fused back together and secured with stainless steel wires. There remained a lot of recovering to do.

Two days down the track Mac took a turn for the worse. His tiny right hand looked mottled, a sickly marble pattern had emerged in the skin of the arm. Worse than that, where the drip line pierced his hand there was a patch of dark purple skin. Gangrene.

The ominous black-purple colour had started as a tiny spot, then spread to form a patch, then sent an irregular pattern of dying skin, creeping up the forearm towards the elbow. Malachy's circulation was clearly failing.

Looking down his supine body we could see the same mottling affecting his right leg, and more frightening still, his right foot was turning more deeply blue. If this continued unchecked Malachy could lose his right foot and his hand.

Some of the medications being used to prop up Mac's heart were causing trouble. Pushing up pressure around the heart was valuable to Malachy, as it helped maintain the oxygen supply to his vital organs. Sadly, the same medications were reducing blood supply to his limbs, as the human body doesn't view hands or feet as vital organs.

Not just loving Malachy as a parent but also having a doctor's understanding, I had felt for the pulses in his dusky foot. I felt a strong, normal pulse in the left foot, but in the right there was no impulse against my fingers. I had drawn the problem to the nurse's attention. Carefully she placed her fingers adjacent to the long bones of Malachy's forefoot and confirmed my worry. The junior doctor was called, further confirming the absence of a feeling of pulsation in the foot. A doppler test was used to confirm there was just a mere trickle of blood working its way to the right foot, in contrast to the corresponding artery on the left, which was bounding along.

The missing pulse would explain why the foot had turned blue and felt cold. Up the hierarchy went the alarm, until the head of this particular team, a smart and pleasant woman ranked by the label 'Fellow' entered the room. The fellow was followed by two less senior doctors and another two nurses. Everyone, Maggie and me included, was keen to see what action she would recommend to diagnose and fix Mac's ailing circulation.

The fellow leaned to place her hand on each foot in turn, lightly furrowing her brow in a show of professional concentration, then straightened to her full height, made eye contact with the assembled throng and said, 'There's a pulse there. I can feel a strong pulse on the right, just like the left.'

Case closed? While this verdict was intended to reassure us that there was no problem, the worry was that if others agreed there was no problem, there would be no action.

The lower rungs of the hierarchy then took turns placing their fingers on the arch of Mac's visibly blue hypoxic foot, concurring that, 'Yes, I can feel a pulse'.

As a parent I felt flattened by the apparent dismissal of my careful observations of Malachy's leg. The difference between the two feet was obvious to a casual observer, but the assessment was reduced to deciding whether it was possible to feel the last faint hint of circulation. The doctor in me was incensed at the system's failure to take a patient-centred view of our well-founded fear. If the family tell you there is a problem, it is foolhardy not to take them seriously. People working in medical systems need to be insightful about the harm they can do by not listening well enough.

The scene reminded me of why I had chosen to work outside the hospital system. Out in the community, being more important doesn't make your fingertips magically more sensitive. Watching a fairy tale of subordination play out over my son's leg frustrated me no end: I was watching *The Emperor's New Fingers*.

The incident, like the earlier distress over the formula milk, and then the central line, is not important in itself, but it is an example of how frustrating it can be to want the best for your child and be thwarted by institutional inertia, powerlessness, and a pecking order. They are examples of how the duress people are under around sick children invades the small details, not just the big picture. There were many small tensions that arose while Mac was suspended in jeopardy. Strain is inevitable given the high stakes involved. In my work I try to stay alert to this. It helps me to judge neither doctors nor patients too harshly.

Subsequent tests confirmed that the circulation was severely compromised.

The dying foot and hand on this day were part of a cascade of events. The main artery supplying blood to the leg, the femoral artery, had been damaged in Malachy's first stay in hospital, demanding that other, smaller collateral vessels make up for the loss. These vessels were not sufficient in his current crisis. And, because a central line could not be placed into Malachy's neck or groin he had to go the more hazardous route of an ordinary drip into the arm. One of the drugs being run in was a vasoconstrictor which narrowed the blood vessels. The drip arm bore the brunt of this constriction.

Nothing seemed to run smoothly for our baby.

We watched, waited, and hoped.

Slowly time rolled on, and with time, other changes were occurring. As recovery of his sternum proceeded, Malachy's heart also did some recovering. His heart's rhythm steadied, and his blood pressure stabilised. Just when it seemed his hand and arm were critically threatened, we had news his heart had improved enough to no longer need the vessel-constricting medication. After more agonising days these changes proved enough to save the limbs. Mac's hand recovered with some scarring. His foot survived. In time, Malachy's collateral circulation would grow to provide adequate circulation for the affected leg. Enough to live and grow.

8

BLOATING AND SLEEPING

*The scientist should treasure the riddles he can't solve,
not explain them away at the outset.*

— Roberto Unger

Remembering Malachy's early years can seem a litany of medical traumas and challenges. As yet he had not developed enough to reveal his personality; in effect he could not 'give back' to those who adored him. There were glimpses of what was to come as his awareness of an audience seemed inherent from the start, but as I reflect on the history, it is clear that they were tough years.

Once we made it home following the open-heart surgery, Mac did have another steady period, but the impact of his life and death struggle on ourselves and the other children was a hidden fact of our existence. Every bit as much as we knew that life had changed for everyone, we were powerless to do anything but walk the road set before us. Imogen had scarcely celebrated her fifth birthday when Mac arrived. Seamus was halfway from three to four, and Niamh as yet a baby herself. Maggie and I were in our early thirties.

From June through to September 1999, we kept on an even keel. There was one serious procedure, with Malachy going back up to Sydney Children's in October for the operation to rejoin his severed bowel. The repair went off without a hitch.

Malachy's infant face had an elfin cuteness about it, often appearing on the verge of grinning, ever ready to be entertained, but could also take on a haunted, frightened look. This would be the face he might wake with, crying in the night, but could also be the frozen uncertainty that accompanied medical illness. The adult equivalent may be the (appropriate) look of terror that says, 'I think I'm having a heart attack' or 'I've just been told I have cancer'. But how does a baby know to widen his eyes, to let them sink in their sockets, and grow still, searching for parental reassurance?

At around ten months Mac became less animated. A stillness crept up on him, as did some fullness in the cheeks, with an unexpectedly chubby evolution of his hands and feet. His propensity to mild clamminess, always evident as if his thermostat were set a few degrees too high, worsened. In January 2000, Mac began to produce soaking wet pillows overnight as sweat exuded from his forehead and drenched his hair.

The medical correlation of this change to a fatter, wetter Mac was that some protein was found in his urine, with dropping blood protein levels. We were advised this was very unlikely to be caused by congestive heart failure (our most feared diagnosis) as heart failure in an infant needs to be very advanced before producing oedema (fluid-related swelling) of this magnitude. So, if it isn't the heart, what is it? It seemed extremely unfair that this tiny child would now have the added burden of kidney disease to carry on those skinny, angular shoulders.

Medical diagnosis being what it is we had to trawl through the possibilities, including the possibility of bowel disease, which would cause him to leak or not absorb protein. Off to Sydney we went to make the rounds of tests and consultations.

The initial cardiology point of view was clear enough: the heart looks good, we need the kidney doctors. Somewhere along the way we encountered a young English doctor, a registrar working in cardiology, who told us of her experiences working with clinics full of people sharing what we sometimes jokingly referred to as 'Malachy's Malady', being survivors of congenital hypoplastic right heart[3]. Most of her patients had had the much talked about Fontan procedure[4]—still a distant prospect for Malachy. The young doctor adopted a bright and optimistic tone, drawing on her experience to advise us Malachy had some reasonable chance of living into his twenties.

Twenties.

After that it was hard to say. There were not enough people far enough past the operation to speak for a future any longer than that. Dying in his twenties was not what we considered an encouraging outlook for our son.[5]

Our journey then took us to consultations, on separate occasions, to two different paediatric kidney specialists, both of whom were known to me and whose judgement I respected. The first of the two requested some more tests and set us the task of waiting for answers, while Malachy bloated and sweated his days away. At follow-up, the second advised with great confidence and a reassuring smile, that Malachy did not have kidney disease, but congestive heart failure. Fear not, he advised, if you treat the failure, the kidneys will behave. He was quite convincing; it was relieving to have a diagnosis, even though it was the one we most feared. I should point out that the medical term 'heart failure' doesn't have quite the extreme meaning you might expect from the usual meaning of failure. It doesn't mean the heart is clapped

---

3 Hypoplastic right heart was Malachy's underlying heart defect. What it means is that the right side of the heart did not develop adequately. The right ventricle was tiny, and misshapen, and the valve opening into the lungs absent. To survive in this condition a child's left ventricle has to be surgically managed to do the work of both ventricles.

4 A surgical procedure used to help manage the circulation of children who have a heart with only one ventricle. It involves diverting the blood returning from the circulation directly into the lung circulation, rather than the usual route back into the heart. The operation is usually done in two separate operations, or stages. First the superior vena cava is diverted (Bidirectional Glenn procedure) and sometime later the inferior vena cava (Fontan Kreutzer completion). Fontan surgery was first performed in 1968 by Francis Fontan and Eugene Baudet from Bordeaux, France.

5 Forty years ago children with single ventricle hearts did not live past infancy. Since development of the Fontan procedure and other surgical advances there are now thousands of people living into their thirties, and one case of a person who lived to age 67 following Fontan surgery.

out, but rather that it is failing to pump well enough to meet the body's demands. Everything got harder as Malachy couldn't pump enough fresh blood forward to his muscles and also had a backlog of pressure pushing fluid into his feet and lungs.

This left us delicately bounced back to the cardiologist—in whose dedicated hands Mac's life had rested several times already—with the need to tell him, 'You got it wrong. There's no kidney problem. It's *your* organ, the heart, that has sent us on this wild chase. Can you fix it, please?'

While diagnosis can be a tricky art form, doctors rarely like to get it wrong so it was no surprise that the kidney doctor's view was met with scepticism, a raised eyebrow and some mutterings of professional rivalry. As a GP, I was no stranger to the specialist tendency to conclude their organ of concern is not to blame for subtle symptoms. What mattered to us was the concession to try the approach suggested by the kidney expert. The concession was gained, a trial of heart failure tablets was commenced, and we settled in to watch for results.

Blood protein levels increased as urine protein levels dropped. The elf returned, the fingers and toes redefined themselves, and the hair began to dry.

Our scrawny, mosquito-like but spirited baby was welcomed back with joy. Our worries were allayed for now, a month or two after the celebration of Mac's first birthday.

As the fluid receded, we were less worried about Malachy's heart, but we couldn't help noticing he seemed to have other less obvious worries of his own.

Maggie and I had always enjoyed the sight of our sleeping children, a joy I had imagined long before ever having children of my own. From time to time I would call Maggie to the doorway of the children's bedroom to soak in the shared happiness of our evolving family life. Whatever concerns keep us older folk awake haven't yet touched the little people, or perhaps they lack the words with which to form their worries. I had thought I would like to go back in time to enjoy that childhood perk, the 'sleep of the just', until we had Malachy. His sleep pattern was terrible.

To this day I want to believe that babies know or remember very little of their 'pre-verbal' life. Can you even have thoughts if you don't have words? Surely the pattern of love and care you receive consistently overrides any ill experiences in a baby? Rationally, I have always resisted dramatic fears about long-term impacts on people from, for example, a brief separation from their mother in hospital or not being able to breast feed. If you can't remember it, it may as well not have happened. Whatever the theories are, my lived experience of Malachy is of raising a baby who cried every night of his life from birth to age two and a half. I recall a baby who woke in distress every night, sometimes suddenly, sometimes with a gradually louder whimper. Not with the hysterical alarm of the 'night terrors' you might see in an older child, but still with vigour and fear.

Malachy needed and responded to a consoling embrace. Maggie strongly believed he was recalling or reliving some horror, that some stain of his medical trauma stayed fresh in his wordless brain. Some track had been laid in which he knew without the filter of language that he had suffered. What does it feel like for a baby to have emergency resuscitation? An unknown world includes a plastic tube that has been thrust into your mouth, down through your vocal cords, you cannot breathe for yourself now, some other unknown entity is forcing air into you through the tube, while another being pumps their fingers up and down on your chest. You are probably unconscious at the time, but how deeply?

Twice in his first three months we had watched as this very scene was played out on the body of our son. We had also watched him suffer the ravages of necrotising enterocolitis, and watched his tortured body edge its way back into life. He'd lived with a 'stoma' delivering faeces through a hole in his side, a hole we had to cover with plastic bags to catch the produce. We watched him recover from having his chest split open by an oscillating saw.

What did he know of all this?

How we responded to this is hard enough to gauge—did we jump with fear too readily, or ignore too much for sanity's sake, or sweat on all the stuff we should have taken for granted? Did we leap in alarm at shadows, and did we pass this onto the child himself? Was he smelling our fear?

But what fears did Malachy have?

Some kind of nightmare woke Malachy every single night. He had worries. We had worries. Maggie and I discussed SIDS, formerly known as cot death, with his paediatrician, Dr de Souza, who explained that should Malachy die in his sleep, we wouldn't be required to undertake the usual autopsy that accompanies SIDS because autopsy is reserved for unexpected or unexplained death. If Malachy died in his sleep, there was an explanation.

9

HUGS

Hugs make you feel psychologically more secure and together.

— Leo Buscaglia

When Imogen was born, I remember floating around the streets near the hospital, hardly aware of time or place. The sensation of a different type of bond, a new dimension to love, was all-consuming. A new creature exists whose characteristics we produced in a Darwinian struggle of Mum Genes vs Dad Genes. There is no courtship nor judgment that precedes this most intense of relationships. One minute the child does not exist, the next they are your world.

Night one of our life as parents found me offering to stay with Maggie until the baby next woke—I would then help her attach for feeding, before heading home for a good night's sleep. Thirteen hours later I had not moved from the spot. I watched every nuance of this sleeping newt, every tiny movement of fingers, perhaps surprised in a dream, every tiny undulation to reassure she still breathed. Never had I been so fascinated by so little action.

Of course, humans form habits and subsequent children can't generate quite the same bizarre and blind devotion for simply sleeping, but the tendency to know every fold of skin, each facial expression, the myriad of tiny genetic stamps either borne out or absent in our child is strong. All parents agonise over the struggles of their children, and in Malachy's life the struggles were of such a scale as to invoke intense scrutiny. Each milestone we feared he would never reach became an emotional touchstone, with poignancy beyond its face value. The accumulated scars and markings of medical intervention and salvation became like a written history on Mac's body.

Buried in the detail of these distinctive features was an endearing feature known to the medical world as 'clubbing'. Low oxygen levels to human hands and feet produce a tissue change in the fingers and toes whose tips become rounded and bulbous, bulging a little to the sides, but also with a swollen pulp and curving of the nail, which loses its usual angle where it meets the cuticle. The tiny, bulbous, blue tips to Malachy's fingers soon became quite rounded and to us, quite beautiful and representative of the boy.

Once he was old enough to recognise this himself, Malachy and his siblings referred to them as his 'domes'. The domes for their part were everywhere. Mac would pick at anything and plunge his hands anywhere. Constant remonstrations from his parents to use cutlery couldn't stop him rummaging through his dinner with those delicately rounded fingertips. These same domes could so often be heard drumming on any firm surface, from regulation tables and benches to his own chest, to any object that potentially resonated.

Before drumming reached the level of conscious activity, Malachy marked himself as rhythmic by tapping away on Maggie or me while being held. To hold, hug or carry Malachy involved feeling a pitter-patter of something on your shoulder, your back, the side of your head. Wherever his hands landed you would feel it: tappity tap tap, tappity tap tap. Was it comfort, reassurance, plain affection, or just a fidgety boy?

To me, I always felt he was passing on love through his fingertips. Those domes seemed to say, 'I am loving being held by you. It's fun staying close like this. Here, have some comfort back from your baby.'

In time his words and actions supported this tactile narrative as he grew to be a young man who loved company and loved to provide company. He loved to be entertained and to entertain. He also remained impervious to the potential irritations of physical touch. Where some people have their moods with being handled, Malachy could be touched, patted, rubbed, tackled and wrestled seemingly without warning at any time, and would never reject it outright.

Breaking one of those parenting golden rules—the one about not comparing your children, for all the psychological baggage they will then have to carry—I must confess that I occasionally put Mac forward as a hugging role model. In his teen years I once drew him to me in demonstration. His impeccable tolerance of parental displays of affection was used as part of an exploration of the more reluctant ways of one of his siblings. On that occasion Mac was tired and heading off to bed, but once accosted, sure enough, he sunk into my arms and just as we parted, faintly I felt it, a tiny, brief, pit, pit pat on my shoulder blade.

Often the notion that I am loved by my children is a subterranean article of faith, rarely spoken, but hopefully assumed. Surely, they will love me forever just for bringing them to life?

Hugging was so apparently natural to our youngest child. Done with just the right blend of firm and tender, without seeming discomforted, neither clinging too long, nor forcing you away unsatisfied or rejected.

Malachy missed no chance to make me feel loved and valued.

10

GETTING AROUND

Aerodynamically the bumblebee shouldn't be able to fly, but the bumblebee doesn't know that so it goes on flying anyway.

— Mary Kay Ash

The constant worry that Mac's hold on life could become precarious was for the most part pushed into the background. Of more concern to us in the day-to-day practice of living was not the existential threat but the impositions of disability. We had little time to pause and recognise how much harder so many simple elements of living were for Malachy, as we were, like him, busy countering the challenges. Mac's surgical repairs, dramatic as they were, did not achieve normal oxygenation. He was well enough to get by but retained the domed clubbing of his fingers and cyanotic colouring, most noticeable in his lips and hands. With cold or exertion, he could look quite purple.

For much of Mac's infancy we toiled with morning medication regimes, sleepless nights, stoma care, delay in reaching both cognitive and motor milestones, a poor appetite, and the need for constant assessment and review. All the while, Malachy hardly grew, and he struggled to achieve the sort of mobility enjoyed by babies much younger than him.

The contrast to his preceding sibling, Niamh, couldn't have been starker. Niamh's motor skills were extraordinary from early infancy. She had once caused a group of adults to burst into laughter with her unexpected speed barrelling down a hallway in her bulging nappy. Her two-year-old legs had a fast enough cadence to bring the joy of pure speed. Niamh had an angelic face crowned by silver-blonde hair and a quiet, independent disposition. If she could do anything by herself, she would. I wonder now whether the fierce independence was simply her nature or born of need while her parents were preoccupied. Like our other children, Niamh showed no signs of resenting Malachy. Maggie and I felt ourselves blessed to have an infant so self-contained who demanded so little of us.

We were occasionally conscious of the way Malachy's travails drew attention away from the other children but remained intent on pouring love into each of them with whatever time we had. Niamh's physical prowess was a source of entertainment for me and her highly developed sense of balance meant I could carry her on my shoulders without any need to steady her by the legs, nor for her to clutch my hair for support. If I lurched one way or the other, her tiny frame shifted accordingly to stay afloat on high.

Niamh absolutely hated being disciplined by her parents. While she was still sleeping in a cot, possibly just two years old, there was an occasion when we had to correct her during an outing. She fumed about it in the back of the family car. When we got home the determined child, barely tall enough to climb stairs, indicated that rather than be sent to her room by her parents, she would march herself there of her own volition. Jumping from the car, she plunged, red-faced and fuming, into the bushes beneath our verandah, scaled the plants, pulled herself over the railing, landing on her feet on the other side, then stomped down the hall. Though startled at first by her wilfulness and then her unexpected ability, we paused to chuckle about how she would indeed have no trouble in fulfilling her promise that she was, 'Going to my bed'. The cot had tall railings and no access stair. I headed down the hall to investigate and was surprised to catch the last impact as she crashed headlong onto the mattress, having scaled the impossible fence of the cot.

'Hats off to you, Niamh,' I muttered under my breath.

By comparison, when Malachy was two, and by all usual measures should be capable of running with ease, he was not yet walking. The much maligned 'baby walker' device struck us as adequately safe and logically worthwhile, and provided the first method by which our precious boy could independently move from point A to point B. This sufficed for a handful of weeks leading up to Christmas 2000 before being supplanted. That Christmas, Mac acquired a plastic tricycle.

The model was a common one for the time, with a red seat, yellow steering console and wide blue wheels. Without much expectation of success, we parked his malnourished bottom on the vehicle, with exhortations to flap his legs for propulsion, and stood back amazed as he shot down the hall chased by his siblings, beaming with delight. This underweight flyspeck of a child, hitherto useless for any form of physical activity, had found something he COULD DO. He could move, he could seek out what he desired, he could show us what he wanted and where he wanted to go. Though we were greatly tickled by the mere fact of his first taste of mobility, what was truly impressive was the dexterity with which he steered and manoeuvred the machine. We'd never seen him be brisk or sharp in his movements, but now he whizzed around the house, darting between people and objects without heed or clumsiness.

The $15.95 or so Santa Claus must have forked out for the tricycle was repaying itself daily as Malachy scooted about to his own great pleasure and that of his siblings. He was a much-improved play commodity, and as he detected how impressed adults were by his skill, he quickly learnt to play up to this—turning his play into an entertainment, and deftly 'working the crowd' with stunts and bursts of speed. It looked harder than walking, but that particular skill remained a distant ambition. Mac showed that gliding on a tricycle required significantly less energy than ordinary walking.

If there had been a hint of emerging baby fat on two-year-old Malachy, perhaps the increased activity that accompanied his discovery of riding was burning that off, for he remained pitifully thin, with a touch of the infant-old-man-prune-face look, and he continued to require full stroller service for any outings.

While Malachy had taken his first steps at around two and a half years, walking any distance, especially if there was a hill involved, remained beyond the capacity of his faulty circulation. In fact, Malachy remained stroller-bound for so much longer than his peers that his speech began to outstrip his physical abilities by some distance. Ten kilograms of weight was a mark at which he stuck well into his third year—the average weight for a one-year-old. Maggie and I were content to make do with the stroller. With the other challenges this boy was busy staring down, we saw no sense in burdening him with expectations of normality.

Mac survived so many challenges by age two that we sometimes referred to him as the 'Boy Who Lived', comparing his resilience to Harry Potter's survival of a blast from Voldemort's wand. Mac was starting to become aware of adult expectations and perceptions. We would often see our boy admired by strangers in a public setting—a pinch of the cheek, a quick, 'Isn't he cute' or 'He's got his father's eyes', and some age-appropriate babbling. Before he turned three, we realised that Mac was entertained by finding himself underestimated age-wise. Unexpected and apparently precocious one-liners delivered from the stroller became Malachy's natural currency. A penchant for sharp repartee would be a defining hallmark of his personality.

The stroller, however, couldn't last forever. As months passed the fun wore thin. Mac started to dislike being marked as less mature than his peers.

Some method of carriage remained necessary. A stroller was still useful on smooth paths in an urban environment, but cumbersome and inadequate on bush trails, long grass, or uneven ground.

Part of the solution was the 'baby backpack', which helped him to enjoy an increased range of family activities, and new sights and experiences. The backpack was terrific for shared exploring. In the end its use would be limited by Mac's weight outgrowing my ability to carry him.

Here lies another avenue by which Malachy planted himself ever deeper in our affection—he could not go anywhere without the manual strain of one of either his parents or his siblings. For me to walk with Malachy strapped to my back meant we shared every step, no stair was climbed without the straining of my legs and quickening of my breath. It was a bonding labour of love, within which I never felt taken for granted.

11

SOUNDTRACK OF INFANCY

If music be the food of love, play on, give me excess of it...
— William Shakespeare

Maggie and I strove to provide the healthiest diet possible for our children, even more so for our youngest who started behind the pack.

In spite of our efforts Malachy promptly established his immovability on the culinary front, having a marked preference for salt rather than sugar by the time he was 18 months old. By three, animal protein with or without noodles trumped any plant material we could present. Highly salted and savoury treats, like olives, salami, and blue cheese, dominated his food choices into his primary school years. When he was five, Mac was admitted to Sydney Children's Hospital for a second Blalock-Taussig shunt operation, where his surprising food preferences achieved transient celebrity. He woke in ICU to exclaim his hunger, and request, 'Sundried tomatoes please'.

As his tastes became more refined, it gradually became apparent that Mac cared not for food at all, really, and he increasingly derived sustenance from the ambience around him, becoming fascinated to engage with people, sights and sounds and ideas, without seeming to need much fuel. Amongst the stimulants dragging him away from bodily maintenance was music.

This was no surprise, really, as each of his older siblings had acquired a 'signature tune' at some early point in life. When

Malachy was approaching pre-school age, Imogen had a nascent passion for piano. By the age of seven, she had already shown a prodigious memory for melody, having once been lured to creep down the hall well after bedtime by the sound of Beethoven's *Symphony Number 9 in D Minor*, or *Choral Symphony* on the TV—a live ABC broadcast of the Sydney Symphony Orchestra performing the work. It seemed to cast a spell on her; she was inexplicably moved and retained a profound love of this symphony from that point on. Imogen found it near impossible to walk past our piano without stopping to play, memorably being photographed once on stopover between her bath and her bedroom, stark naked, with a tangled mop of wet hair, her towel spilling over the edges of the piano stool. Largely self-directed, even as a toddler, Imogen had declared she wanted to do things 'ALL MY BYSELF' (sic). Emotions ran deep in our eldest daughter, who would occasionally become inexplicably maudlin. In tears she would proffer a lost teddy as the unlikely source of her sadness, crying after bedtime prayers: 'I miss Curly'.

Seamus's signature had more of a folk-rock flavour. We discovered that when restless, he settled best into sleep rocked in time with Bob Dylan's *Forever Young*. He was initially a naturally calm and accommodating infant, having happily been duped into pushing Imogen around on a tricycle by the time he was able to walk. Seamus had had his own medical drama as a one-year-old, having series of seizures out of the blue that required treatment with phenobarbitone for almost a year. Thankfully, the problem disappeared without a trace, but it had served to demonstrate what it was like to feel the grip of parental fear. Seamus became more animated after Niamh's birth, showing what would become a lifelong tendency to thrive on a receptive audience, as well as spending his third year frustrating us with exhibitions of sibling rivalry directed at the new arrival. Seamus kept his words to himself, barely talking until such time as his first words rolled out in fully formed sentences. By the time he was four, Seamus had earned Imogen's respect for his emerging intellect, having given her unsolicited help with her readers before reaching school age himself.

Niamh, for her part, didn't seem to notice the clobbering she received from Seamus on arrival. She appeared resilient but did need more coaxing off to sleep than we were accustomed to with the others. The most potent remedy became rocking back and forth in her stroller, using the edge of our lounge-room carpet to create a rhythmic bump in time to her signature lullaby: Rachmaninov's *Piano Concerto Number 2 in C Minor*. I would frequently be lost in the rumbling movements of the tune, still rocking her after she was deeply asleep. As far back as I can remember Niamh was independent beyond her years, adamantly refusing parental help with packing for excursions or holidays. I would have to find room in the car for assorted bags and cases which to a fault contained everything we would have packed if we'd been allowed.

Once Malachy emerged from the maelstrom of his medically menacing start to life, he too picked a signature tune, squawking at age two from the back of the car that he wanted to hear, 'Bah–Baaah!' This referred to a tune better known by its opening four chords: Ba-Ba-Ba–Baaah (G,G,G,E!), Beethoven's famous introduction to his *Symphony Number 5 in C Minor*. Given his troubles with sleep, this tune was frequently deployed for Mac's comfort. As soon as he was able to demonstrate his personality, Malachy became an entertainment for the others. They laughed at his precocious taste in music, his natural comic timing, and his willingness to let them amuse themselves at his expense.

This little family of individuals enjoyed plenty of age-appropriate children's music over the years, happily pointing to fingers and toes in time with The Wiggles' entreaties, and later embracing the musicality of The Hooley Dooleys. By the time Malachy started listening, there was some pressure on these old favourites to give way to the future. The older guys could still enjoy bouncing along to the children's bands and also felt old enough to enjoy a burst of sentimentality about the songs they'd learnt only a couple of years earlier, but increasingly they were finding more interest in other music. They liked the albums Mum and Dad played when our 'Wiggleometer' pointed to ENOUGH. Snippets of Ben Harper, Tracey Chapman, U2 or even Jackson Browne's *Stay* were evoking sympathy from the crew—much to our relief after seven years of *Dorothy the Dinosaur* and *I'm a Slug*.

Amongst our friends, Mac became known as something of a Midnight Oil fan, and certainly something about the iconic Australian protest rockers struck a chord with him, as it did with our other children. Seamus, in particular, loved to wile away the hours combing through music with Malachy, part mentor, part accomplice. At times the two boys seemed to have a language of their own. Each of the children impressed us with the quality and diversity of the music they would combine onto CDs. They rightly could claim entitlement to some credit as music editors. Somewhere in the house we can probably still find such family classics as *Roc 'n Roll with Sea Sea*, *Mac's Rocn Celekshen* or similar eponymous title.

The Red Hot Chilli Peppers' album, *Californication*, was released in June 1999, and became a favourite household soundtrack, adding a contemporary rock zeitgeist element to the mix of alternative, classic, indie and singer-songwriter fare that held sway at our place. Malachy was just passing his first birthday as this growing musical consciousness took off.

When he turned three, Mac commenced at our local community pre-school, and naturally attracted some attention for his frailty and his relative disability; but there was no form card by which staff could measure the precociousness of his personality. He may have been just like any other child, but blue.

One day Malachy overheard one of his teachers disciplining a peer at pre-school. Mac looked at her, perhaps surprised by the atmosphere of conflict, and tunefully blurted, 'Hey, Teacher, leave those kids alone...'

This may not have turned out to be too pretty, but by the teacher's report, this is how it ran…

'What did you say?'

'Hey, Teacher [etc.]'

'I thought so. Where did you get that from?'

'Pink Floyd.'

'You like Pink Floyd?'

'Yeah.'

With the young woman thus disarmed, a lucky child was no longer in trouble and a pre-school teacher was on her way to succumbing to this most engaging of infants. By the next week Malachy was describing to us the locket worn by her that contained the secret photograph of her late brother who had died in a motorbike accident.

Who was this child for whom death carried no taboo, and grief became a chance to meaningfully engage? What place has any three-year-old caring for the feelings of a woman in her twenties? Contrary to logic, part of me believes that Malachy understood the beguiling impact of his curious emotional bravery.

12

GLIMPSE OF THE MAN

The deeper that sorrow carves into your being, the more joy you can contain.

— Khalil Gibran

After the extreme drama of Malachy's first three months of life we made a few changes to try to ease the strain and approximate normal family living. Maggie reduced her teaching load to part-time and casual, while I made sure I protected my Fridays off work for parenting. The medical challenges kept coming, but we took them in our stride.

There was the abdominal surgery when Malachy was six months old. This was the operation to rejoin the bowel where it had been cut to form a colostomy in the week Mac was born. In the absence of serious complications, I hardly remember this operation now. It added two more long pink scars across the middle of his belly.

Mac's puffing up with heart failure at 12 months had been worrying at the time, but once the right medication was introduced had eased without incident.

At 18 months, Malachy had another catheter, or coronary angiogram, without cardiac arrest, collapse or catastrophe. The angiogram confirmed what we knew of Mac's disordered anatomy but suggested there were no critical changes afoot.

Maggie and I worked hard to keep up with Mac's needs, but also tried not to let this dominate our home life. The period of relative stability allowed the other children to concentrate on being children, and Malachy to set about growing and maturing.

Malachy's bedroom contained an inexhaustible supply of soft toys, a legacy of his hair-raising newborn period. Many friends and acquaintances, and even some strangers, had found themselves confronted by the drama of Malachy's struggle and, lost for suitable words, had shown their concern in the form of a menagerie of giraffes, koalas, puppies, owls, and teddy bear after teddy bear Each one was attributed a name and a personality, and a whole secret life that would be acted out on or under Mac's bed, on the floor, in the chest of drawers, and spilling out into the hall. From time to time the motley collection would also raid other rooms around the house.

As Mac grew older, the cuddly toys were joined by plastic toys: figurines of endless variety, from the known and familiar (Power Rangers, Ninja Turtles and the like) through Lego people, farmyard animals and movie characters, to unnamed incidental finds— unusual alien characters, space travellers, and once famous sports figures. Each of these also had an inner life of their own, fitting into the broad category of team good or team evil. It was never clear which side of this grand historical contest Malachy favoured.

Day after day, hour after hour, Malachy covered his room with battles and sagas involving the innumerable characters. No story was too complicated to try relaying to his uncomprehending parents. I am sure that in the heat of these battles Malachy was forging the stories that would propel his narrative style in years to come. The constant practice at plot twists and near-miss escapes reflected and built on an agility of mind. The tales he would go on to write unfolded at the same breathless pace as these early battles.

Maggie and I counted our blessings that this child, so limited in physical ability, had the consolation of such a fertile independent imagination. He asked very little of us in the way of input into his games. His imaginary world was replete without parents.

61

In November 2002, Malachy was nearing four years old. His cousin Lucy, who is also Malachy's godmother, had included him and Seamus in the bridal party for her wedding. Our two daughters were also dressed up for the occasion, objectively the prettiest flower girls I'd ever seen.

In what may have been a formative experience, Malachy was a dashing figure in his dinner suit and tie. This was the first time he'd worn a suit, his typical scruffy, quirky cuteness being kept in check by the formality of the garb. Maggie and I shared the glow of parental joy as we watched our progeny pose for a beautiful set of images, nestled against a backdrop of Sydney sandstone on the shores of Pittwater.

Malachy's infectious grin started out well but fatigue eventually got the better of him and the other young models. The children started to get tetchy as the photographer strove for perfection. Increasingly, the poor man wrestled against the hunger of the younger members of the bridal party who broke away at the first hint that shooting was complete. Malachy sighed his relief and moved into the throng of guests, whereupon he was pounced on by more camera-wielding adults. Wearied by the posing and pressured by the throng of adoring relatives, sweating in the warmth of his dinner jacket, Malachy broke free of the pack and sought my hand.

'Dad, let's go for a walk.' His eye roll emphasised the desire for escape.

'Okay, where will we go?'

There were limited options, the reception being perched between a cliff face and the water, and the path out requiring a climb beyond Malachy's ability. We moved towards the only free space which was a boardwalk along the foreshore between the venue and the daunting stairs. The dusk had deepened enough that the glow of some bordering path lights now sparkled against the backdrop of the water, illuminating the path and the rough charm of the yellowed sandstone to our right.

'Dad, I just need some fresh air and a break! Will you talk to me?'

As we made quiet progress along the boards the sound of water gently lapped against the rocks below, and from a nearby boat pattered a flap of canvas. All else became still as the murmur of the party faded behind us.

'How are you enjoying the wedding, Mac?'

'It's good, Dad, but a bit crowded. I just feel like hanging out here for a while.'

I said something in reply, but sensed I was losing my audience. His hand in mine became still and a hush descended as we perched against the fence at the end of the walkway. I looked down at his still, faraway face and saw the calm drawing of his breath. Malachy looked deeply satisfied, as if reflecting on completion of some grand achievement.

In the quiet, alone with my son but in proximity to so many loved ones, emotion flooded in. What a struggle it had been to reach this point of peaceful solitude in the company of a child I feared would never know peace.

As I looked across the water, I had a clear sense of what he must be feeling. The moment hung, time perfectly suspended while our senses soaked in the damp air, the fading pink light of the clouds, the gentle slap of unseen waves, and the happiness of two people. Happiness, and a glow of profound contemplative joy. Can a three-year-old even feel that?

'Isn't this beautiful, Dad? The path and the lights, with the water. So perfect. It feels as if this place was just made for us to enjoy.'

Something profound inside that three-year-old boy made him impossible not to love.

Four months later in April 2003, Malachy's cousin Alice was married. Malachy had just celebrated his fourth birthday. The reception was again by the water in a small cove known as Shelley's Beach. The venue is accessed by a wide shared footway, popular with joggers, walkers, riders, and all manner of outdoor enthusiasts.

As the wedding crowd neared its destination, we found the going hindered by a group of young skateboarders. In baseball caps and oversized clothes, the gang of boys spilt across the path, nonchalantly dismissive of the well-heeled guests who stepped around them. The vibe they gave off had a hint of aggression, and the young children gave them a wide berth.

Except for one of them. Arriving at the reception and finding Malachy absent from the group we looked back down the path to see him in earnest interaction with the skater boys. Recognising no boundaries of age or class, heedless of potential menace and possibly needing a rest to catch his breath, Mac had stopped to talk to the lads. It turned out he'd admonished them for intruding on the thoroughfare and they'd fired back at him. He'd proceeded to give smart answers to their repartee, apparently smart enough to win them over. I hurried back to gather him in my protective arms. By the time I reached Malachy, he was enjoying a demonstration of the boys' board tricks, handstands, parkour and other physical skills.

Seeing that he was safe, I put a polite lid on my exasperation.

'Mac, we're all waiting for you!'

He tilted his disappointed gaze at me.

One of the lads, cap backwards, looked my way and asked: 'Dude, is he your kid?'

'You got a pretty funny kid, mister. Can we keep him?' said another.

'It's okay,' I joked back, 'I'm pretty happy to hang onto him for now'.

I smiled and took Mac's hand. As we turned to leave, the youths entreated Malachy to, 'Come back over when you get bored, mate', and the like.

Mac, in his four-year-old way, explained that he'd 'got them in trouble' for impeding the path, but agreed to 'let them off if they could impress' him with their stunts.

'Mac, you could get yourself in trouble with kids like that. I didn't know where you'd gone.'

'They did some pretty good tricks, Daddy.'

'I'm sure they did, mate.' I shook my head in wonder.

Mac's array of toys had the advantage of requiring far less maintenance than pets, which was helpful as our family record at keeping pets alive was poor at best. Birds, fish, rabbits and guinea pigs struggled to live to a healthy age at our place.

Maggie would sometimes find herself with unexpected 'me time' once the older children had left for school and Mac had retreated into his fantasy world. One still, winter morning, she sang to herself, breezily cataloguing her thoughts while tidying the kitchen, and came across the last of our goldfish floating dead in its tank. Free of the demands of school-age children and with Malachy tucked away in his room, Maggie decided to flip the fish out the window where it could later be scooped up for burial. She grabbed his clammy little tail and, with a flick of her rubber-gloved wrist sent him off to the lawn below. Turning back to the room, she was startled by four-year-old Malachy watching from the doorway.

Malachy turned his face upward, head tilted, with a quizzical expression on his face. He took a breath and asked an unexpected question: 'Mum, are you going to throw me out the window when I die?'

13

HOSPITAL FAMILY

Human beings have enormous resilience.

— Muhammad Yunus

Maggie and I consulted a new cardiologist, Stephen Cooper, with Malachy, just after he turned five. Malachy had been quite steady for the preceding two years but had become increasingly short of breath in early 2004. Mac presented as a little boy who had outgrown his oxygen supply. The little clubbed domes of his fingertips sounded a warning; through January they were becoming a deeper shade of blue. So too were his cyanotic lips as his breathing grew more laboured. He needed more oxygen, and he needed a plan for keeping up with future growth and change in his body.

Dr Cooper recommended two things: a fact-finding catheter and more heart surgery.

Neither of these were straightforward.

As it stood, Malachy's anatomy and underlying complications prevented a safe, successful catheter. The problem was his blocked inferior vena cava (IVC)[6], through which a catheter would normally pass.

The choice of an operation was not simple.

---

6   The inferior vena cava is the major vein returning blood from the lower half of the body into the right atrium, ready to be pumped to the lungs. It is the target vessel for the final stage of Fontan surgery, the Fontan Kreutzer completion. A blocked IVC reduces the usefulness of this final operation.

Consideration was given to a heart transplant, but the expert view was that Malachy's left ventricle was good enough not to warrant replacing the whole organ. Transplant had other problems, including needing to move to Melbourne for treatment, requiring a lifetime of immune suppressive medication and being hampered by a shortage of donor hearts. Another option was to try to perform an operation called a Bidirectional Glenn shunt[7], but the safety of this could not be guessed at without first performing a catheter.

After consultation and investigation, Drs Cooper and Nunn advised that the best path forward was for installation of a second shunt, mirroring his existing one. A new Blalock-Taussig shunt would solve two problems. The extra connection to the lungs would give Malachy more oxygen and it would also allow passage of a catheter through the shunt to complete the follow-up angiogram. For this operation he would have to have his chest opened again, not through the zipper on his sternum this time, but with an incision through the back between two of his ribs.

We felt confidence in our advisors, so the plan was agreed. Malachy was booked to go back into hospital in March; we braced ourselves for the next hurdle.

Inexplicably, Malachy always maintained a favourable view of hospitals and their staff. While Maggie and I wondered whether his nightmares arose from the hospital traumas he had been through, we couldn't avoid noting in him a little frisson of excitement that attended his admissions evidenced by the constant cheeky smile he wore in hospital, pushing through whatever fearful or sombre thoughts were attached.

After working in both paediatric and adult hospitals, I had often mused that the latter had a lot to learn from the former. In 1994 I was a junior doctor when I first walked the wards of Sydney Children's Hospital (then known as Prince of Wales Children's

---

7   The Bidirectional Glenn procedure is the first stage in Fontan surgery. It aims to divert the blood returning from the upper half of the body, through the superior vena cava (SVC), to the lungs rather than the heart.

Hospital) and was struck by the chirpy, 'playschool' atmosphere. This contrasted with the bland décor and sombre atmosphere of the adult equivalent. Regardless of the suffering within the rooms and theatres of the children's hospital, the effort to amuse and comfort the patients sprang from every wall, curtain, desk and ceiling. A child could not lie on a bed without discovering pretty diversions: a Disney picture, a luminous set of planets, a painting in primary colours. That sick adults miss out on all of this says something about an emotional retreat or a fear of some unspecified discomfort that we acquire with age.

As Mac's parent, some credit must accrue to whoever set this cultural foible in motion, for the intended sense of welcome and wonder was not lost on him. Personal resilience, cup-half-full optimism, and a social disposition positioned him well to benefit from the amassed goodwill of the staff, the decorators and their many allies.

Cheerful images, even happy memories, spring to mind. I can picture Malachy tickled with delight as a nurse introduced him to one of the computer games accessible through the *Starlight* console. I see Mac's hospital-gowned body frail and cyanosed, his purplish lips brimming with joy as the young nurse took him through a humorous explanation of the rules and risks of the game. Mac was entertained by and bonded with the staff who attended his bedside, not just trusting, but also interested to engage, to laugh and be laughed at. It was every bit as consoling for me as for him to feel the personal care that so many people brought to their work with our boy.

One enduring memory our family can laugh about is that of Malachy's contributions to the Starlight Channel as a four-year-old. This channel was part of an in-house TV system at The Children's Hospital Westmead, compered by Captain Starlight and accomplices, who would at times take requests by phone that were screened live throughout the hospital. Inspired by I know not what, Malachy took to the use of his female alter-ego, Sarah, for his dealings with

Captain Starlight. Sarah was a collaborative invention of our four children who took excessive delight in dressing Malachy in the girls' outgrown dresses. Malachy responded enthusiastically to the mirth of his siblings, enjoying the in-house celebrity Sarah brought him. The other three thought themselves hilarious with this creation, so they were in fits of laughter around the bed whenever Malachy phoned through a request in character to the Starlight Channel.

At first the Captain was dubious about the quivering voice of this young girl, but with repeated acquaintance, no doubt felt guilty he had allowed himself to be amused by her strained, unusual voice. The sounds produced in the struggle with whatever chronic malady Sarah suffered were quite unfortunate. Having ultimately passed this level of identity check, Sarah was able to entertain viewers with quirky and challenging requests of the compere, and at the same time brighten up the bedside vigil of his siblings and parents.

For better or worse, Malachy developed such familiarity with the hospital experience that he had an unwritten list of preferences that could run from mundane choices of pyjamas and clothing to unexpected technical matters like anaesthetic preference. In keeping with the special care taken with paediatric patients, one of the services offered by anaesthetists is to be sent gently off to sleep by the 'magic wind'—a whiff of anaesthetic gas, bypassing the terror of intravenous cannulation.

During the consent process for one of his operations, we went through a gamut of benefit versus risk, potential complications, etc., prior to signing the forms. Before pen went to paper Malachy requested to know how he would be put to sleep. 'Will I have a needle or the gas?' he wanted to know. 'If it's the gas, I don't want the operation.' Here was a boy requiring in advance that he has the dreaded needle. Malachy found the smell of anaesthetic gas unpleasant and for that moment this was his greatest concern in the approach to major surgery.

Unexpectedly, given its far-reaching reputation, another hospital pleasure for Malachy was the food. The quality of the mass-produced food in a hospital setting is possibly the most maligned of the services on offer and often cited as the explanation for weight loss after a long stay. Malachy, however, lit up about the food. The arrival of a meal brought a satisfied smirk to his face and an enthusiastic reception for the wheeler of the trolley. He may not have eaten all that was presented, but there was no doubting the ability of this ritual to help him feel special. He was fed like a king, while the signal to others was clear—look on in hunger or leave to find your own meal. I loved the pleasure he took in such a small consolation.

The rest of us did have our own hospital food experiences, too, including through our stays in the Ronald McDonald House facilities at both Randwick and Westmead. One of our trips to Randwick gave us the remarkable, once in a lifetime pleasure, of eating No Problemos for breakfast. It was a Simpsons'-themed cereal that was produced very briefly in 2003, becoming our favourite of all time before it disappeared from the shelves. Its existence coincided with a catheter procedure.

It wasn't really the discovery of No Problemos that made Ronald McDonald House special. It was being surrounded by other families who shared the terrible bond of having a desperately ill child. The families each experienced some variant of the strange displacement our life had acquired. There would be many childhood moments like this, institutionalised moments. The group kitchen, the shared resources, the hostel-style rooms and the endless, tense waiting periods all became normal life to our children who just adapted, innocently. Simple joys in a complicated setting.

While stays at the hospital involved drama and trauma, they were also usually times through which we were intensely supported. Family and friends would arrive with flowers, food, games and puzzles—all manner of thoughtful contributions to help us pass the time, preserve sanity and maintain nutrition. So the hard times are happy times, too, for me. Times when people make their love more obvious.

I suspect the children share this ambivalence about those days. I hope all the treasures designers have planted around those hospitals touch the children in the way they planned. I hope some trace of the magic of The Faerie Garden lingers to enrich a quiet minute, or that some happy reverie is sparked by Captain Starlight, or some familiar playground equipment. Maybe one day a child of mine will break into a smile remembering the pretty sculpture of the child with cancer we found on a walk through Westmead. Maybe the clown doctors will be remembered fondly during a circus performance, or a stroll through a remote village might remind one of them of the hidden pagoda courtyard, their first glimpse of Asian garden design. I hope so, because so often the hospital was where we needed to be.

I have often been asked how we managed to juggle the needs of ourselves and four young children through this period with so many frightening interruptions to our life. The most obvious answer is that I don't know, that we managed because we had to. Friends and family helped support us through umpteen mini crises. We learnt a lot about the right time to turn up with a meal. One vital cog was our local Nanny and stand-in-grandparent, Colleen, known affectionately as Colly, who was a constant presence through Mac's early years, serving up good humour, cackling laughter and baked dinners to our household.

14

HAVING A BALL (FOR THE CAUSE)

You may never know what results come of your actions,
but if you do nothing there will be no results.

— Mahatma Gandhi

Malachy's heart disease exposed us to a vast world of hidden needs. Childhood heart disease scarcely registered in the public mind but afflicted and killed more Australian babies than any other single condition[8]. Despite this, it did not give a sufferer automatic qualification for a Health Care Card. The forms for a doctor to apply for a child disability allowance have three pages of 'accepted disabilities', with not a single mention of heart disease. Very little is known about how to prevent heart malformations and most of the treatment for serious conditions is palliation rather than cure. Well-meaning people often exclaimed to us how amazing it is what medical science can sort out these days, implying on the basis of no specific knowledge at all, that Malachy would 'be right' soon enough.

Each of the major children's hospitals in Australia have a Ronald McDonald House facility for families to use while their child is being treated. When we first needed this type of assistance,

---

8   This figure does not include those otherwise healthy babies who die as a result of birth complications, which account for 53% of newborn deaths. Once the delivery is survived heart disease is responsible for 7% of deaths under the age of 1, as compared to sudden infant death syndrome (SIDS) accounting for 3%. (Australian Institute of Health and Welfare date, 2017)

while Malachy undertook his initial open-heart surgery, the accommodation was not available to us because Malachy didn't have cancer. The best we could do was find lodgings in the Parent Hostel where our other children, aged two, four and five, could not be housed with us. The hostel provided a room with a single hospital bed and a fold-out on the floor. Major heart surgery wasn't recognised as causing significant family upheaval in the same way that cancer treatments were.

As heart disease in children simply didn't register on the radar of public concern, until they had an affected child, a family did not realise that childhood heart disease meant frailty, weakness, pain, shortness of breath, repeated life-threatening events, surgical wounds, scars, and severely traumatised relationships.

Maggie and I were confronted by how little was known of the suffering of the people we met fighting against their child's burdens of disease, incapacity, and premature death. We were meeting people who were absolutely shocked to land on a desperate medical rollercoaster they didn't know existed. There were almost no dedicated services and little access to information.

Each major treatment centre had scrambled together only the beginnings of a 'Heart Kids' social support network. There was a coffee morning here or there, a support meeting in a hospital room where you could discover there were other families like yours. It felt simply wrong to find so little on offer to guide people through the vast and all-encompassing challenge of coping with this disease. This was something just not right in the world.

It took a few years before the tentacles of need, obligation, grief and fear of an uncertain future drew first Maggie, then me, into the world of support and advocacy.

HeartKids NSW in 2002 and 2003 offered coffee mornings at the hospital and a chance to meet and learn from other parents who had lived the journey with their own child. The committee meetings were by and large social support gatherings providing an opportunity to be with others who understood your version of suffering, in all its loneliness, fear, powerlessness and serial trauma. Meeting other parents provided a ray of light in those darkest of days. It meant so much to us that we, in turn, couldn't ignore the urge to share the benefits of with others.

So, we became involved with HeartKids. It started as a trickle, with Maggie meeting the wonderful people who were the backbone of the existing support group in Sydney. This meant having to make a six-hour return journey to Sydney for a one-hour coffee, or a three-hour committee get-together. Committee meetings were usually at night, so on those days it would be midnight before the rest of us saw her.

As Maggie became more involved, she started to meet a wider network because HeartKids NSW was making links to similar small groups elsewhere. If there were so many sufferers, where were they? Where was their voice? At that time there were early whispers of the idea to link all the tiny hospital-level gatherings to form some larger entity. The parents of Heart Kids were still scattered widely and were lone voices with a faintly heard telegraph system crying out to know others—to know whether there was hope for their child, to know what was next, to find some help.

Maggie was bitten by the glaring needs of these people. Her enthusiasm to make a difference became infectious through 2003 when she roped me in to help out. I thought it should be simple. The statistics were so compelling, the cause so straightforward, surely the doors would just fall open—I thought no one could resist the logic that the greatest killer of children should get the greatest funding.

As time revealed, there was a quagmire of barriers to helping the children and their families. Maggie and I felt that there was so much 'low hanging fruit' that could be picked to care for heart kids and their families such as having heart disease recognised as a disability, getting better access to accommodation, and having funding for support workers.

But it was harder than we imagined. We found ourselves part of the movement to grow the cause. Heart Kids needed a strong and nation-wide organisation to champion their cause. and we were on hand when the first steps were being taken to form HeartKids Australia.

Involvement in HeartKids increasingly entailed unknown personal costs, however. Maggie and I had to consider what neglect our children might suffer as more of our time was given over to the organisation, its fundraising and campaigns. We agonised over the balance between our own children's needs and the net effect if nobody cared enough about serving the great needs of so many other families. We tried to balance role modelling activism and dedication against domestic availability. As a sufferer, or as a sibling, do you need your parents focused on you or will your life be improved by seeing your parents out in the world, trying to be part of the solution? We were unsure whether our children would gain more from sharing Malachy's struggles than they would lose through missing out on the normal freedoms of childhood.

The competing demands were challenging, but necessity was our master. We felt every bit as bound to keep faith with the HeartKids struggle as to keep on being parents.

The love of our fourth child demanded it.

When it came to it, Malachy was every bit as engaged in the cause as his parents. Wherever we went he was also bound to go, and vice versa. Our voluntary involvement included having a hand in marketing. Faces were needed for brochures and pamphlets, quotes for articles, pictures for magazines and voices for radio.

Handsome little Malachy with his cyanotic lips and winning smile found his head popping up in different promotional spaces. Amongst press clippings and other memorabilia, we have kept copies of a brochure informing people about HeartKids, with four-year-old Malachy smiling in the sunshine with the caption: 'Meet Malachy from NSW, new discoveries are yet to be made to fully address his condition'.

Having a ball (for the cause)

With encouragement from Cecily Waterworth, then president of HeartKids NSW, Maggie volunteered to turn her hand to fundraising, since her teaching obligations were now much reduced. She rallied her local friends in Nowra who got behind an event entitled the 'Heart Kids, Malachy and Friends Ball', the first large formal fundraising event of the organisation's history.

The ball took place in March 2004 on the Eve of Malachy's fifth birthday, with his shunt operation looming. Nowra came out in force to support both us and the cause, and also to use a brilliant excuse to party hard. The locals mingled with HeartKids' members from far and wide, along with a range of celebrities who donated their time, marshalled by Maggie's schoolfriend, Josie O'Reilly. Wendy Harmer performed a comedy routine, Josie put on a show of improvised comedy with Andrew O'Keeffe, and the funny and amiable James O'Laughlin acted as compere. Our local paediatrician, Dr Mark de Souza, leant some gravity to the fundraising by speaking about the medical difficulties confronted by children like Malachy. The event ended up involving 500 guests and raising close to $60,000.

It also showcased Maggie's ability to rally people to the Heart-Kids banner, propelling her into the inner circle of the NSW branch. A few months later she was taken on as a manager, becoming HeartKid's first paid employee.

15

CHEST TROUBLE

'I'd like Malachy to have another chest X-ray in two weeks.'
— Dr Cooper

While Maggie and I had both grown up in Sydney, neither of us felt wed to it as a permanent home. Maggie's parents had moved to Cootamundra, in the Riverina, and we had friends scattered through the farmlands, so rural life held no great fears or stigma for us. Nowra had answered our needs as a place to set up base once children were in our sights and General Practice had become my calling. The town has a wonderful mix of proximity to mountains, river and beaches, as well as reasonable proximity to the bright lights of the city. Rural General Practice had a range of pull factors being community-based and wholistic, and the telling push factors of not being hospital work, and of not involving city traffic.

From day one we had been very happy in Nowra, joining the practice of Dr Col Shepherd, the father of an old schoolfriend. The way the local community rallied to our support following Malachy's dramatic entry into the world turned Nowra from a nice place to live, into a home for life.

Contrary to the evidence of our sedate country life, Maggie and I hung onto a belief that we were adventurers. Twelve years earlier we had both resigned our jobs, Maggie after four years teaching primary school and me, having completed my one-year medical internship. We'd bought an old campervan from some English backpackers, loaded it with camping gear and our mountain bikes, and headed out around Australia for a year-long road tripping adventure. The vibe of that year, 1992, had lived on inside us, as some kind of bug we hoped our children might catch.

At the start of 2004 we had spent just over a decade submerged in the breeding and infancy phase of family life. Our yearning for adventure was coming to a head and we were optimistic and determined to make it a great year regardless of any obstacles. But now we found ourselves staring ahead at a patchwork of competing interests.

The older three children were busy working their way through primary school, calmly absorbing the dramas thrust upon us by 'Malachy's Malady'.

Maggie's Nowra ball was taking a tremendous amount of work and planning to realise.

Malachy was getting bigger, and in some ways more independent, but needed to have his next big operation.

Before the need for a new shunt arose and ignoring the other potential barriers, Maggie and I had made plans to embark on a Great Aussie Adventure, namely, to haul all the children off camping in the outback for a whole school term, teaching as we rolled along. Second term was the target—taking off in the Easter holidays, returning in July for term three. The timing had seemed perfect as the ball would be done with in early March and the school term would finish at the start of April. The dates would coincide with optimal weather up the coast and into North Queensland. The children were all coping well with school and seemed unlikely to fall far behind while absent.

The problem with our plan was Mac's operation, booked for March, stuck right there, smack in between finishing with the ball, and hitting the road.

Excited as we had been in January about our travel plans, our hearts sank as we looked at the logistics. Dr Nunn said a seamless recovery would take only a few weeks, but it was clear that any serious complication would rob the family of our planned odyssey. We lowered our expectations and put off making a Plan B. The ball and the operation gave us plenty to focus on, so the trip would be surrendered.

As it turned out luck and skill combined in our favour. Mac breezed through the operation in flying time, waking from the procedure a new shade of healthy pink. Graham Nunn was pleased. We were thrilled. Mac left hospital after just a few days with less strain on his heart and a better circulation. The internal restructure was expected to meet his needs for many years to come.

Surprised by the speed of Mac's recovery, Maggie and I leapt at the opportunity to put the adventure back on our calendar, booking ourselves out of work and signing the children off school for the next term, and the holidays either side. From Easter to July we would be on the road with a borrowed camping trailer. Along the way we hoped to instil in our young tribe a love of adventure and a sense of freedom from the conventional strictures of a workaday life. That holiday was burdened with great expectations.

Leading up to Easter, a week before our scheduled departure, Maggie held Mac back from preschool one morning, as he felt a little short of breath. Maggie took him down to my workplace to see his GP, Adam, who ordered an X-ray. Mac's breathing got gradually heavier as the day progressed. The X-ray confirmed the complete collapse of one lung, submerged in a large volume of fluid, which must have leaked from some part of the operation site.

Maggie took Mac on the urgent drive to Westmead for admission and treatment while I was left to sort out work and the other children. The path forward was frightening but seemed simple enough. Go to Sydney to see the surgeon at the hospital. Have the fluid drained. Patch up the drainage hole and voila!

What transpired was a harrowing experience. The next two days were bad enough to stand out even in the battlefield of Malachy's lifetime of travails. There was no bed available on the ward, so Mac was left in an emergency cubicle. The staff were stretched, and after reviewing Malachy, assured Maggie he could wait the night to be definitively managed on the morrow. Their confidence didn't stop Mac's chest from steadily succumbing to the weight of fluid pressing on his right lung. He went from bad to worse. Maggie was horrified to have a child vomiting relentlessly in the neighbouring cubicle. There was only a thin curtain to stop Mac from catching whatever was being thrown up next door. Forced to sit up all night in a plastic chair, Maggie desperately tried to find a way to convince the Emergency staff that Malachy needed more help.

Sometime after midnight the initial reassurances gave way to shock when they recognised how grave things were getting. Malachy could scarcely breathe and would almost surely succumb if he caught the vomiting bug from the next cubicle. Dialling up the amount of oxygen in his mask was barely keeping him stable. A chaotic scramble through the middle of the night led to welcome news that Malachy was being put on the operating theatre list for the next day. The staff placated Maggie with the news Mac would be first on the morning operating list. The only preparation required was to fast from midnight, ensuring an empty stomach en route to theatre. The early morning hours dragged on.

By the bright light of morning Mac was hungry and breathless but at least buoyed with relief that repair was at hand. As 8 o'clock passed by, however, it was evident that he was NOT first up on the list; Malachy's starvation would need to be a little further prolonged. The morning, and the fasting wore on. As 10 and 11 o'clock rolled on he was NOT second on the list as it turned out, either. Dehydration began to assert itself and better information about exactly when the surgery would be become elusive. Someone had botched the organising. Malachy's heart raced and his blood pressure plummeted as worsening dehydration was added to his weight of symptoms; the fluid collection pressed more heavily on his straining lungs. One false reassurance followed another as Malachy became drier and sweatier, a deeper purple colour suffusing his parched lips. Nonetheless the Emergency staff didn't seem to comprehend how vulnerable his situation was.

Maggie's desperation approached crescendo, until she was forced to explain fortissimo Malachy's past cardiac arrests and his rapidly worsening listlessness. Then he reached the brink of collapse. Suddenly aghast at their own misjudgement, the staff sprang into emergency mode. Apologies were offered while the alarm was raised. Trolleys surged back and forth, curtains were flung open and the crisis response enacted.

Mac was rushed to the operating theatre. A silicon drain mounted on a large bore needle was inserted through his side, between two ribs, into the cavity around his lung. Surgical pain gave way to relief, as straw-coloured fluid poured out of Malachy's chest, flowing through the silicon tubing, into a sterile plastic container.

The little silicon tube and its collecting vessel were to become our constant companions for many days as the build-up of fluid stubbornly resisted the expected drying up. Approaching two weeks, our travel plans were once more receding as the doctors debated the next step. Was a further operation needed to tie-off a leaking vessel or would Mother Nature step up to the plate and seal off the leak. It was unclear whether this was leakage through the material from which the shunt was fashioned or from an incision through a lymphatic vessel. Lymphatic vessels are part of the immune system, carrying the pale-yellow lymph fluid around the body. They don't tend to heal as well as blood vessels because the lymph has no clot-forming platelet cells.

Malachy looked vulnerable and pale but made no complaint about this drainage tube poking into his lung, or about the adjoining apparatus he was forced to carry everywhere. We wheelchaired him all around the hospital, and around our temporary home at Ronald McDonald House. All the while the fluid stayed constant, and the surgeon hovered at the ready.

The complication dragged on through Easter, into the time we had planned to be far away to the north. The older children had some unexpected consolation for their displacement, receiving a large bounty of Easter eggs at Ronald McDonald House. There was so much donated chocolate that Niamh later asked whether, should Malachy require another operation, it would be possible to schedule it for another Easter.

Preparations were made for another bout of surgery. Then virtually overnight, without any intervention, the fluid dried up. A day later the drain came out and Malachy was deemed fit for discharge. The advice from the cardiologist was that we check for complications with a follow-up X-ray in two weeks' time but that there was only a small risk of the lymphatic fluid re-accumulating.

16

FRASER ISLAND

'This is the worst day of my life.'
— Malachy Frawley

In two weeks' time we were 1,720 kilometres from home, or 20 hours and 35 minutes' drive north, in Gladstone, Queensland.

Given the time we had lost to Malachy's lung collapse, and his weakened state, we had to weigh up whether fate was telling us to make new plans. Maggie and I certainly had some misgivings and some extra ache over our vulnerable fourth child and were mindful of the need for the check-up X-rays. Nonetheless we had built up hope that our Great Aussie Adventure would be a formative and bonding experience of childhood.

So, we cast aside the noise and worry and bundled all six of us into the car with all the other necessary baggage. Our mission was to create lasting memories that would help define their childhoods as happy, a secure base to console through inevitable challenges.

We had long held that holidays are made memorable by the disasters they entail but doubted this road trip could out-disaster what we'd been through in our domestic life. Stowed somewhere in the vehicle with us was a subtle fatalism, a bit of 'Who knows how long we have as a family?' I wasn't prepared to admit this to myself.

Amongst the threats to be wary of on our journey were disastrous acts of nature such as a tropical cyclone or tsunami; anthropogenic disasters such as a road traffic calamity or sunken boat; and fearsome encounters with wildlife—disembowelling by an angry cassowary for example. For the most part these were avoided, but there came a day that presented us with Malachy's perfect storm; his three or four most hated elements rolled into one package tour.

That day was always going to prove difficult for our youngest child, who had suffered a bout of diarrhoea in the days leading up, weakening his already challenged body and taking the edge off his enthusiasm for anything beyond a quiet day at the campground.

Our long-imagined destination was Fraser Island.

An iconic part of the Australian must-see tourist adventure, Fraser Island featured in political struggles to save it from obliteration by sand miners in the 1970s, then was feted for its surviving colony of purportedly pure-blood dingoes, then has been intermittently notorious for attacks on the unwary by these same creatures. The island is an adventure wonderland with pristine world heritage elements for your contemplative side, and ample challenges for camping and survival skills, as well as ocean fishing opportunities that have passed into legend.

Unpacking these elements as they apply to Malachy, the 'wonderland' breaks down into four-wheel-drive tracks, sand, water and heat. Malachy was a victim of travel sickness. The real kicker for him was rough or winding roads. Fraser Island's sandy tracks were both rough and winding, with unpredictable jolts of acceleration and deceleration. I watched as Mac's face drained of colour and took on the cheek-bloated look that warned of impending vomit. He started asking, 'When do we get out of this bus?' The answer was that we couldn't stop while on the sandy track as any other vehicle would not be able to pass, so we must press on to the open beach.

Optimistically, I felt relieved when we finally pulled up adjacent to an outcrop of coffee-coloured rock on the expanse of the beach that forms the eastern coast of the island. A nauseated, bedraggled, disheartened and already complaining Malachy alighted on the sand and started to walk away. Then he stopped.

Sand. Sand. Sand. The whole of Fraser Island is made of sand. Sand, which forces people of normal fitness to work a bit harder, but for Malachy was a torturous stress test. In normal circumstances Mac bravely tolerated walking on flat surfaces and even small inclines, but usually ended up being piggybacked once he reached his paltry limit. He could never manage sand. He dreaded it. Quite aside from its retarding softness, beaches almost always slope, so whenever Mac had been to the water's edge, he would have to climb a hill to escape, on sand. Every step on sand required an effort at the limit of his capability.

The only thing we knew that sapped Malachy's oxygen faster than walking on sand was swimming. He couldn't do it. After a brief stop on the sand, the next stop on the tour had been chosen because passengers had the chance to swim down a permanent watercourse towards the ocean. As everyone else stripped to their swimming costume, there was Malachy, unable to take part in this next activity, a would-be relief from the heat of the day. Mac sat on the sand, sweating in his jeans, blue as the ocean, crumpled on the boundless plain of sand, defeated and cranky.

As the elements converged on the hapless child there came a moment when our attention also focused on his squatting figure, astride of a small mound alongside the tour bus. The clouds of misery looked set to burst just as he sensed an audience, and we briefly apprehended Malachy was gathering to an announcement. He declared loudly: 'This is the worst day of my life'.

Most other days were much better than that one. Some of our hopes for the holiday were probably more targeted to the older children who would be old enough to remember it in greater detail than Mac.

Niamh was turning seven that year and would entertain us while scaring herself with her bike-riding feats around the trails wherever we went. Slight in build, she was nimble and tomboyish, and remained very self-contained, striving to match her older siblings, forever seeking permissions beyond her years.

Seamus at nine, as dark of hair and skin as his sisters were fair, was a quiet child. He usually thought things through before speaking and had shown such ability at school as to occasionally be spotted by his mother left at the helm of a classroom, reading to his fellow students while his teacher was on an errand. He had spent much of his time over the years mucking about with his neighbourhood mate, Mikey, whom we had caught up with en route through Goondiwindi.

Imogen, at eleven, was almost always best of friends with Seamus, and was a very capable all-rounder. She excelled in schoolwork, sports, and creative endeavours, and also delighted in establishing games within the family. The others loved her pretend school which she conducted with a toy chalkboard on the side veranda of our house.

One of my fondest memories from the trip is the afternoon we spent at Trephina Gorge, in the red desert of the East MacDonnell Ranges near Alice Springs in Central Australia. Maggie and I took a path up one side of the gorge, on a relatively safe walking path, with Niamh in tow and Malachy riding on my back. We left the others to explore the precarious terrain, aware it was a developmental step for them to have such freedom. As Seamus and Imogen scaled the uneven rock columns of the opposite side of the gorge the acoustics proved exceptional. We chuckled to each other as we overheard an excited exchange between the two senior members of our brood.

'Wow, Shea, this is so cool. I can't believe Mum and Dad let us do this by ourselves.'

'Yeah, it's pretty high, hey.'

'Yeah, I can't wait to tell my friends we did this dangerous climb by ourselves. I hope it's not too hard to get down!'

As we plunged further into our adventure, such pleasures gradually erased the pain of Malachy's claims to a rock-bottom experience at Fraser Island.

17

THE ADJUSTMENTS

I am still making order out of chaos by reinvention.
— John le Carré

Our gang of six experienced countless marvels in what I still believe was the best term of learning the children had in their school careers. I base this on no evidence whatsoever, not helped by the children's unanimous claim that the only lesson they remember was my explanation of the cycle of the moon, delivered at a camp table, with the sunset over King's Canyon as our backdrop. Admittedly this is the only formal lesson I can recall too.

I have been lucky enough to make several forays into overseas travel and find it fascinating how much you learn about a place by being there and gathering the stories endemic to the country or culture you encounter. Nothing brings home the history of colonial conquest quite like seeing the varied architecture of a series of different conquerors lining the streets of a single town. To my repeated amazement, having made roughly two laps of Australia in my life to date, it's no different travelling around our own country, a place I have known since birth and think I can feel in my bones.

The first time I went 'Up North' in Western Australia I was constantly wondering, 'Why weren't we told?' For example, when Maggie and I encountered the legend of Pigeon Jundumurra, a dramatic and significant resistance hero of the Kimberley, we had to make a trip all the way to Tunnel Creek to even hear of him. Australia's geological history is fascinating, but for some reason it barely reaches the attention of those of us raised in its populous cities. The history of human settlement dates back at least sixty thousand years and holds numerous lessons for those disposed to learn. Colonial history is riddled with stories of failed settlements, with forlorn pioneers perishing for want of simply asking the locals, 'Where is the water around here?' As climate change and soil degradation march on unabated, we learn more all the time of the complex stewardship of Australia by its traditional owners, and how we could profit from their accumulated wisdom.

Our family odyssey would ensure we came to appreciate the wonder of an ancient culture that enabled people to survive in what looks like vast infertile deserts and overwhelming heat and drought. We also chipped away at our ignorance of our vast continent's geography. As an example, we stumbled on Queensland's massive, wondrous, Undara lava tubes. We had never heard of these huge cylindrical caves, the residuum of enormous volcanic eruptions which spread across northeast Queensland, a geological age ago. Similarly, I had no idea that the 'alien landing' capital of Australia was, as the signs claimed, at Wycliffe Well, a resting point now known in our household for the worst-tasting water in Australia. We were even ignorant of North Queensland's endangered cassowary—a magnificent giant flightless bird—before we saw the local signs that warned it can disembowel you with its talons. We laughed at warning signs depicting tourists covering their tender bellies with backpacks to fend off the avian beasts.

As we pressed on with the trip, our hero's inability to enjoy sand, water and physical exertion was overwhelmed by these unexpected delights, and also some more famous ones. One early morning we watched platypodes (or is it platypuses?!) at play, fossicking in a pristine waterway high in the clouds of Eungella. We soaked in the grandeur of Uluru, King's Canyon and the Wilpena Pound. We walked in dry heat through the ancient domes of Kata Tjuta, marvelling at the bright red colours and the unyielding harshness of the desert. Malachy and the other three were thrilled by the underground settlement of Coober Pedy, with its tales of pioneering lawlessness and its unique opal-riddled landscape.

Other native fauna to highlight the trip included saltwater crocodiles in the Daintree, wedge-tailed eagles feasting on carrion at the roadside, and oodles of koalas and kangaroos. We even included a trip to the zoo built by the late Steve Irwin. One animal story to pass into family lore is the barramundi fishing expedition. Four children each caught a fish, two of which we ate for dinner, while the other two were passed back into the water. By a feat of parental mathematics, each child knows to this day the fish they caught was firstly the largest of them, and secondly, was one of the two that ended up in our bellies that night.

A small personal odyssey for me added poignancy to the journey. One place we visited was the Darling Downs town of Toowoomba, where my father had grown up. Dad was born into an Irish farming family in which his father had the exalted position of eldest son. The full benefit of this was not realised, as my grandfather had been disinherited of the farm for reasons lost in time. Dad grew up to be the first university-educated person in the history of his family, being granted a scholarship to study medicine in Brisbane. I had spent several summer holidays visiting the Queensland branches of my family as a child. When we pulled up with the trailer outside the Frawley family home in Hume Street, I enjoyed a lovely burst of memories.

Further on in our trip we camped somewhere just north of Cairns. At the campground there was advertising for joy flights to Thursday Island, a tiny island in the Torres Strait, making a tiny dot on the map just beyond the Australian mainland's northernmost tip, the Cape York Peninsula. I contemplated making the flight as this island had further sentimental value to me. My mother, born into an English family with both Royal Navy and British spy (MI 6) pedigrees, had not been content to pursue her nursing career in the safe familiarity of London. Instead, she'd flown to the distant colony of Australia, intent on helping improve the lives of Australia's Indigenous people. Finding Sydney completely swamped by its European invaders, with a relative shortage of original inhabitants, Liz had answered an advertisement in a local paper to disappear into traditional Indigenous lands in the remote north.

After landing on Thursday Island, no doubt radically unprepared for a place so foreign to her leafy Surrey upbringing, there wasn't much to resemble the comfortable life she was accustomed to. The tiny village community that included just a handful of non-Indigenous people led her into the company of the Island's only doctor—a young red-haired surgeon by the name of John Frawley, who was posted to the island to begin paying back his Queensland government scholarship. The rest is the history I enjoyed relaying to my children around a far northern campsite in 2004, though I didn't end up taking the joy flight.

So much was packed into that three-month period that by the time we returned home the trip had proven a certifiable success. Maggie and I were both refreshed. We had met our need for adventure and had built a happiness bank for future withdrawals.

Returning to the grind of daily life quickly threatened to make such a bank useful. For three months we had only had to answer to the immediate needs of our nuclear family. Malachy was in a world where the five of us could tailor every activity to be acceptable to him. We walked at his speed, or carried him, or avoided the most physically demanding adventures. Our gorgeous older children lived with these adaptations all the time. The freedom of the road allowed us to be available for Malachy's every minute.

Once we were home the comfortable nest could not be maintained. We couldn't protect Malachy from the strains of normal day-to-day life.

Malachy had two godmothers—his cousin Lucy and Maggie's friend Jenny, who lived across the river from us. Jenny was very engaged with Malachy, often going for outings or activities with him, and he loved spending time at her place. Days at Jenny's usually involved some cooking, at which she excels, and Malachy had fun both joining in the craft and eating the produce.

One 'Jenny day' involved Malachy having a brief stay with her family while we were away for the weekend. They had spent a day on the town, with a meal and some shopping. Jenny arrived with Malachy back at our house.

'G'day, Mac, hi Jenny. How did you go? Have you had a good time?'

'Yeah, Mum.'

'We had a lovely time. We've been around the shops and walked through the street. It was a really busy day. Malachy might be a bit tired.'

'I am a bit.'

Malachy's slump into a chair was evidence of his fatigue.

I made the customary offer: 'Can I get you a cup of tea, Jenny?'

'That would be lovely.'

We three adults adjourned to the lounge room with our cups, out of earshot of the children.

Leaning forward, Jenny said, 'Maggie, I don't know how you do it'.

'Do what?'

'Do anything. Go out, walk around. I had no idea how hard it is. You have to do everything so slowly.'

'I guess we're used to it.'

'He really doesn't walk very far. It was exhausting just getting up the street. It's lucky he's easy enough to carry, but I don't know how you get anything done.'

Most of the time we were scarcely aware of this. Rarely, one of us would have an outing with the other children, *sans* Malachy, and be amazed how quickly we could arrive somewhere by foot, guiltily revelling in the freedom of movement such as a dart across the street against the lights, takings stairs two at a time, carrying nothing, looking ahead to our destination. A truth that needed to remain unspoken was how much fun it was not to have to wait, to hold your speed constantly in check, to worry for every slight incline, every hurdle, every crossing. Outings with Malachy were a labour of love we never begrudged, but a *labour*, nonetheless.

So, although Malachy was master of the tempo of our family life, requiring restraint of sorts at every turn, it didn't stop the children pursuing their sport, each of them taking up many opportunities in that field. But the nature of play within the nuclear family was constrained by the invisible hand of Malachy's limitations. Artful accommodation had become second nature to all of us.

If we didn't go to the beach, or if the fun park was off the holiday agenda, or we didn't kick a footy at the oval, no one complained. My remembered childhood full of sport, of Mum calling six resistant boys and a girl in from their backyard footy as the light disappeared from the sky, was the template I started with in my career as a parent. It was a template I quickly forgot as circumstances moved it out of reach. Filial love involved numerous tiny acts of omission, of missing out.

Niamh, Seamus and Imogen show no resentment. You can reason through what effects numerous little acts of kindness and accommodation might have on a growing person. As a parent you fear the worst for your children; resentment and 'carer burnout', craving for attention and reward. What we hoped for in our children is what we mostly saw rise to the fore: compassion and tolerance, resilience in the face of challenge, and a deep understanding of disability and marginalisation. I confess I greatly enjoy the sin of pride as I observe in my adult children a strong sense of justice. Was this in their nature or a product of the leavening effect of Malachy?

The impact of so much adjustment around disability in the family network is something I have pondered. From a rational point of view, it is as incalculable as most of the 'Nature V Nurture' questions. It is known from anecdotal reports and from studies of the numbers that severe illness or disability in a child increases family breakdown. Our luck may have been to have this particular child, with this particular malady, which had the opposite effect of rallying people around and drawing us closer.

As to the effect on Malachy, how can we guess what might have been? Who would be brave or mean enough to ask him what it feels like to be forever making people wait for you or soften their play so that you could join in, or carry you because you're too weak?

Buried in the lifetime of cheerful coping, the determination to be himself and not recognise the barriers ahead, lie countless unseen hours of pondering and wondering, and coming to terms with the harshness of fate.

Rarely would such thoughts make a public appearance.

Malachy was sometimes agelessly profound, but later that year, settling back into the rigours of school, the child hidden inside revealed itself. Heading off to sleep, with his mother at his side for the nightly ritual of tucking in, after a prayer to his guardian angel, he spoke of misgivings.

'Mum, I know it's good to be a Heart Kid, and I know I'm special, and all that, but sometimes it gets pretty hard.'

'Yes, darling.'

'So, I've thought about it, and I don't want to be a Heart Kid anymore. Someone else can have a turn now.'

Stooping to place her arms around his bony back, holding his warmth to her, her head buried on his shoulder, a tear ran down each of Maggie's cheeks.

'Oh, Malachy, I wish it worked like that.'

18

ACTIVIST AND OBSERVER

As my sufferings mounted, I soon realised that there were two ways in which I could respond to my situation: either to react with bitterness or seek to transform the suffering into a creative force. I decided to follow the latter course.

— Martin Luther King Jr

A year after the Nowra ball a cover story on *Who* magazine describes Angelina Jolie as 'Every Woman's Worst Nightmare', while inside, from page 40, four families, including our own, tell of the 'traumatic but often inspiring journey of raising a child with a heart disorder'. The story goes on to explain that Maggie was at this point the NSW Manager of HeartKids. *Who* relays to the readers Maggie's report that Malachy 'has been very conscious of death; there have been lots of questions about it including, "Am I going to die before you?"'

In working for HeartKids NSW, Maggie had left teaching aside to wrestle with the source of our family pain. The *Who* article quotes her, 'There'll be times when he finds it tough in the playground'. But there, as if to contradict her, in glorious colour, crossing the double-page spread, is a family portrait, in long lens, so our hero is seen in sharp focus; Malachy not yet five, head tilted cheekily, with a half-knowing glint of inspiration for his audience. He senses something special about his message to the world. Arm-in-arm, the other five of us are bit players, our range of emotion open to interpretation. We all have to accept whose show this is; the boy has intuited it is him that people want to see.

Malachy felt himself to be special by virtue of belonging in HeartKids so was willing to help fashion the message to others, that being a Heart Kid is hard; you are different from your peers, you face challenges they may never know or understand, but you are nonetheless cool. Such aged wisdom inside that skull held on young puny shoulders, but held for the most part so gracefully, so lightly.

Maggie and I did whatever we could to support Malachy's interpretation of his heart disease in favour of special, rather than disabled or excluded, but his willingness to put effort into the work of HeartKids was more than a response to our input. Malachy cared for people. He had started to get to know a range of Heart Kids and felt the intense bond of shared suffering. He loved his friends and wanted to model a positive attitude and do whatever else he could for their cause.

Malachy was particularly motivated following his first experience of a HeartKids Family Camp. This was a part-funded getaway to camp-style accommodation at a beach suburb near Newcastle. It was the first time any of the Frawleys had been away with a group of families selected by virtue of having an index case of childhood heart disease.

Maggie and I were able to feel a communal sense of knowing that marked the gathering. We all knew disaster-parenting through lived experience. Children's heart disease doesn't obey the socioeconomic fault lines of smoking and lifestyle-related adult disease, so the gathering though small was diverse. There was one family in particular who stood out to our children. Their three children were effusive, unrestrained, noisy and chaotic, starkly contrasted to our retiring brood. The middle child was a fierce amazon; leader of the pack, charging her way around the camp tirelessly. Malachy was duly impressed by her bravado, her individuality, and apparent oblivion to the approved gender stereotype.

That evening, better acquainting ourselves with our new friends, we unpicked the 'who's who' of each family, the stories often starting by identifying which of your children has heart disease, of what type, and what does it mean in terms of treatment and the like. The infant amazon it turns out was the affected child in her family—the Heart Kid. This was unexpected from my perspective given her physical presence around the playground. For Malachy this was unregisterable. Non-comprendez. Not true. No way. A Heart Kid who can run and swim and fight was a previously unimagined world. Affliction was a matter not just of type, but also of degree.

After the camp, Malachy entered a pensive stage. This first encounter with a large group of other Heart Kids had clearly thrown him. Among other things, he hadn't previously conceived of a Heart Kid being able to charge around with such abandon. Sense needed to be made of this, but for now it was clearly very affecting. We hoped for the better.

The topic was rejoined some weeks later, when six-year-old Malachy was the one to raise it. Maggie was working in her home office this day, surrounded by HeartKids' paraphernalia. Her role included awareness-raising, so she had a hand in the marketing: posters, logos, brochures and the like. A familiar image to us and to many families involved with HeartKids, was the stunning picture of Maddie, a gorgeous young girl from Victoria, her round possum-like eyes staring serenely out of the poster. The innocent beauty of the child's face captivates the viewer, who can also see the child wears no shirt, but instead on her chest wears the great rent of a surgical scar, the signature of recent open-heart surgery. The bone of her sternum has been sawn through then rejoined. A still-bloodied suture line is framed by the tails of her long white-blond pigtails. Surgical gauze hides a drain site, and a few white sticky strips help support the wound. We may not have drugs that make you go bald, but heart surgery images sure can pack a punch!

'Mum, I've been thinking. That was really good what we did with those other families. I think it would be good for me to spend more time with other HeartKids.'

Maggie, who'd sensed Mac's need to talk, turned to make eye contact.

Then, with index finger raised, eyes cast to the wall: 'Mum, I think I'd like to meet, say…' he paused, 'her'. Pointing to our poster of the captivating Maddie.

Precocious as ever, we suspected he'd taken a fancy to the pretty face in the poster hanging by the desk, but unquestionably, the seed of recognition of a common destiny with other Heart Kids was germinating.

The day Malachy had endured Fraser Island I had been slow to recognise the burden of heat, travel, sand and water on him. I gained deeper insight one hot summer day during another family camping experience. I had, what my children teased was an annual tradition—a torn calf muscle acquired playing twilight cricket. I was having great trouble walking with my leg heavily bandaged to prevent any painful twist of the ankle, so was perfect company for Malachy, in my lame state I shared his reluctance to plunge into the discomforts of camping. He and I lodged at home while Maggie and the others pitched their tent on the sandy grounds of Bristol Point, part of the Booderee National Park at Jervis Bay.

We were invited to join a large group of friends swimming at the nearby beach of Greenpatch. In 36-degree heat, Malachy and I met the others at the campsite, a short walk from the beach. The able-bodied crowd tore off to join the fray, leaving the two of us a long way behind. Sweating profusely in the searing heat, we started making our way along the track at 'Mac Speed'.

As I paused from time to time to steady myself, Mac shared the pause to regain his breath. The trees up ahead which I would usually breeze past seemed frozen in time as we inched along the sandy path. Gradually the birds that customarily skip past or avoid the crashing sounds of human walkers made themselves more present to us. Little brushing sounds near the track took on a fascinating hue as our senses aligned themselves to our surrounds. Tiny blooms on the fronds of native plants shifted into focus.

We both felt it, but it was Mac who put words to it. 'You see, I love this, Dad. By walking slowly, you see so much more.'

We shared the time in discussion of this: how beautiful are the unnoticed elements most people rush past in daily life, how fertile is the world in minute treasures and quiet pleasures. I was in Malachy's world of hidden wonder.

As the absence of a sense is said to enhance others, so was Malachy disclosing an enhanced power to draw more from a simple moment, to observe the physical world more closely.

Being as impressed by super-heroes as most boys his age, Mac wondered aloud whether he had stumbled upon a new superpower? The power of 'Disability Induced Hyper-Observation'.

Maybe!

If this was a superpower, Mac had a sense of how he would like to put it to use. He liked to help people, and he liked to write stories.

MALACHY'S MAGNUM OPUS

Esteban Devereaux's Adventure

Chapter One

— Malachy Frawley 2013

Esteban Devereaux was sitting in the middle of the street. He just sat there, cross-legged and breathed deeply. The warm sun was beating down on his wavy brown hair, and glinted in his mismatched, green and blue eyes. As he sat there he realised he probably looked homeless. He was wearing mismatched shoes that matched his eyes, red threadbare pants and an old, frayed light-brown woollen jumper. He was surrounded by houses that all looked exactly the same which was strange because they were all plain and boring. He would have thought the council would have realised this but instead they just kept on building, expanding their lack of creativity.

'Hurry up, Esteban,' called Valdus from up the hill. 'You've been catching your breath for three minutes now!' Valdus was Esteban's close friend. He was pudgy with astonishingly rosy cheeks and straight, orange hair. Standing next to him was Esteban's other friend, Firnen. Firnen was fast and strong, he was the opposite of Esteban in every way. His weirdly dark hair fell over his eyes so that no one knew the colour of them because no one had ever seen them. Esteban had no idea how Firnen could see, but somehow his eyes seemed to be able to see through the black curtain which was his hair.

Esteban stood up and slowly walked over to them, struggling his way up the large hill. 'Come on,' Firnen said, 'You're as slow as an ant!'

Valdus looked at Firnen quizzically. 'Ants aren't slow.'

'Yes, they are. Look at how many we've overtaken.'

'They're just small.'

'Well, I mean he's covered as much ground as a human in the time that an ant would.'

'But ants aren't really affiliated with speed; more just size and strength.'

'Fine, you're as weak as an ant.'

'Ants aren't weak.'

'Alright, **now** I know that you're trying to be funny.' He looked at Esteban. 'He's being funny isn't he?'

Valdus sighed and slumped, clearly having given up on the debate. The boys continued up the road for a good one hundred metres, but it was only a matter of time before Esteban sat down on a brick wall outside someone's house.

Both Valdus and Firnen groaned, 'Again? We'll never make it to the top of the hill!'

Esteban shook his head, 'What is so important about getting to the top of the hill?'

'It's part of your training,' Firnen said.

'Ah,' Valdus said, 'don't you mean his recovery?'

'Whatever. I just like to refer to it as training 'cause it's more manly.'

'As if it isn't already manly enough. Have you even SEEN his scar?'

'Yeah, it's **damn** manly!'

They continued up the long hill, stopping at regular intervals, having some banter, and then continuing on. Half an hour later they made it to the top and looked down the road. Then they turned and gazed out at a beautiful orange sunset and basked in the sheer awestriking beauty of it. Suddenly that painstakingly long walk all seemed worth it. The wheatfields below them were blowing gently in the wind, making nature's very own Mexican wave. Esteban thought that he could not believe something as beautiful as this was soon going to be replaced with more uncreative, boring grey houses. It seemed a crime to him that something as plain as the bland, grey buildings behind him would be replicated and put in the very spot he had spent an hour of his life struggling up a hill to see. The boys turned around and stared down the road.

'See that, Esteban?" said Firnen. 'You've looked death in the eyes today!'

'Been there, done that,' said Esteban, much to Valdus's amusement.

'Yeah,' he said. 'Several times.'

'He's best mates with death now,' said Firnen jokingly. 'It's more like, Oh, hey Death, listen man, I'm good. Why don't you just go back to your wife and kids. I'll be fine, don't you worry. Just come back for me in seventy years!'

Esteban laughed. He found Firnen extremely amusing and always laughed at his raw stupidity, like he was doing right now.

'Let's go,' he said, 'that's my exercise for today'.

They began the long descent down the road in the receding light of the setting sun. Esteban was about to have another rest but instead Firnen just picked him up and kept walking.

'Hey!' Esteban said, 'what the heck are you doing?'

'I'm bored of resting and your house is only a few metres away, so I'm carrying you.'

Esteban stopped struggling, and just relaxed. Soon they made it out of the grey suburbs and to the more colourful part of their town, where Esteban lived. They stopped outside his house and said their goodbyes to each other as the sun dipped out of view and darkness overcame them.

'See ya, Esteban,' said Valdus. 'You know, you've really achieved something today. You really conquered your heart disease.'

Esteban smiled. 'Thanks, Valdus.'

PART 2

PRIMARY YEARS

the laws of the jungle

19

A WISH UNDER DURESS

'I have an idea, but I don't think you'll be able to do it.'

— Malachy Frawley

We had known some people over the years who had been touched by the work of Make-A-Wish which does wonderful work granting wishes for children with life-threatening medical conditions. The main beneficiaries tended to be children with cancer while those with heart disease were not as easily recognised by the charity.

So, it took a little bit of work to convince Make-A-Wish that Malachy was a legitimate recipient of their interest, with Maggie and I needing to garner certificates indicating that Malachy's life could be greatly shortened by his disease. Of course, all the while we hoped this was stretching the truth.

An experienced volunteer from the charity, Max, came to our home to interview Malachy and his siblings, to determine whether he had any desire to experience something in particular. Many children have touching stories of meeting a hero from sport or entertainment, or visiting a long-dreamed about theme park or natural wonder. Our advice was that Malachy was to decide, though the others were allowed to be present as guides, or perhaps merely as a courtesy to them. They had some ideas of their own— Disneyland polled well—which turned out to be Mac's preference as well. Unfortunately, Make-a-Wish had age constraints around overseas travel, so a trip to meet Daniel Radcliffe was out of reach for the same reason. Both these choices would have delighted the whole of family and had been discussed beforehand.

As those options stalled, Mac adopted his 'genius at work' persona and alerted the gathering: 'I have something I would want, but you won't be able to do it'.

'Well, try me, you never know,' responded Max.

'Nah, it's okay. It'll be too hard.'

'What's your idea, Malachy?'

'Well…' (pause for effect, or maybe thinking time) 'I want to direct a movie'.

'Noooo, Mac,' was the chorus from the others.

The wish-maker then continued, 'With me starring in it, and writing the script'.

Okay, now it emerged: Malachy didn't really want to meet a hero, or a star, he wanted to BE that guy. The seven-year-old walked from the room, casting a 'Wait a minute' glance over his shoulder to the others.

Tainted by experience, and in the process of arriving at realistic worldviews, the three older children were instantly aware of the unlikely nature of the project and conscious, too, of the many possible failures this could entail. Waiting for his return, they feared Mac had no perception that there is no audience for the mighty talents of precocious seven-year-old wannabe stars. They well knew Mac's stories were madly vivid in the mind of their creator—if not ultimately coherent to the world outside—were dramatic and frenetic in a stunning way, if not always sustained by narrative logic.

Two minutes later Malachy returned, bearing notebooks and loose sheets full of writings, penned in secret, surprising everyone with a fully formed action tale ready for translation from novella to screen script.

'So here is my story. Can we do it?'

Having no yardstick by which to judge the sanity of the impish, blue-lipped child before him Max replied, 'I can't see why we couldn't try'.

Some scoping discussion ensued, with the conclusion from the day's exertions being that Max would go away and nut out a few ideas and see what Make-A-Wish had to say. He named some celebrities with whom they had dealings who might be available for casting and the like, before taking his leave.

Meanwhile on the home front the Wish met with a mixed reception. There was laughter, to be sure. It had been quite entertaining to have Mac stun his siblings with this previously undeclared ambition. His quirkiness was roundly appreciated, but it seemed he may have gone the way of black comedy; our hero was unaware of his own glaring inadequacies. At the same time there was excitement—under the teasing and bemused head shaking, it did seem clear our little boy really wanted this. Something strong inside him would not be denied and in the quieter moments I am sure I was not alone in feeling the infectious pull of his imagination.

Malachy had a movie title ready to scale up for the big screen: *Max Martly and the Fantastic Group.*

Doubt was expressed about the film-readiness of Malachy's handwritten stories, the intelligibility of his plotting and the magnetism of his central characters.

The doubters included everyone but Mac.

20

DEEPER INTO HEARTKIDS

*If the world were merely seductive, that would be easy. If it were
merely challenging, that would be no problem. But I arise in the
morning torn between a desire to improve the world and a desire
to enjoy the world. This makes it hard to plan the day.*

— E.B. White

Malachy's early primary school years measured approximately
from the time of our campervan adventure to the unveiling
of *Max Martly and the Fantastic Group*, was a period of constant
challenge and demand. Time has dimmed my ability to feel the
acuity of intensity and drama, but the history remains, written
into the lives of numerous colleagues and fellow travellers. All
our lives are marked by our involvement with childhood heart
disease, etched to different depths in some kind of proportion to
the effort expended.

These years involved a time in which HeartKids could seize
the opportunity to have a greater profile and capacity to fundraise,
advocate for and serve its families, or accept that this involved too
much change and strain, and remain content to act as an emotional
support group. Thankfully, we and many others sensed the time
had come to step up. Waiting was not an option if we wanted to
help many of our children, but even with tremendous effort it was
uncertain what could be achievable in their lifetimes.

Whatever energy or time we had left over from providing normal family life in our home was swiftly consumed by the myriad tasks of building a unified national charity. Most parents have times of exasperation when they wonder why on earth they took on the unexpectedly hard role of raising children. Four children is deemed a large family in affluent western societies, and we were not immune to the temptation to make sure our children weren't missing out. Our tally of activities to be taxied to and fro included drama classes, music lessons (piano, violin, drums and clarinet), soccer, rugby, basketball, little athletics, art classes and gymnastics. This ordinary peak-hour children's business had gaps for respite, typically while young people were at school or preschool, or once they headed off to bed.

The gaps filled.

Looking ahead at our unrelenting commitments Maggie's and my need for adventure snuck up on us every now and then. I checked out some websites spruiking the idea of medical locuming in Ireland, the home of ancestors on both sides. Teacher exchange in Canada caught some attention. Maggie was keen, but the expense, and the current demands of our family life, volunteer activities and work made it nothing more than a pipe dream. At work I was training junior doctors and had a large patient base that needed to be looked after. Maggie was flat out. Still, it was fun relief to talk up the idea of getting away. It kept alive the spark of our belief in adventure.

Maggie's days became submerged in tasks which were frequently pressing. Her role as state manager grew and grew. Sometimes a special event was approaching with deadlines, or a contact had fleeting availability. Sometimes a gap or imperfection in our current practice was just so glaring it demanded prompt redress. Much of what needed doing depended on cooperation with others, sometimes in Sydney, sometimes interstate. Many days Maggie drove early to Sydney, only arriving home well after dark. Her small home office was crammed to overflowing with promotional materials, brochures, and a range of fundraising paraphernalia.

The demands couldn't be kept to the hours available. The drag of duty into the home office spilt ever more into family time. It was a constant presence in our evenings, weekends, and other spare time.

It wasn't only Maggie. I had long maintained the practice of devoting one day a week to family life. Once the others were all at school, I had devoted my day off to Malachy, whose life expectancy was uncertain in the early years. Through the middle of the 2000s I began to share in Maggie's contribution to HeartKids NSW, first accepting a role on the board of directors, then as one thing led to another, taking on the inaugural Chair's role with the new national organisation, HeartKids Australia.

We organised and took part in HeartKids conferences, board meetings and seminars, in Perth, Sydney, Melbourne, and Adelaide. HeartKids work took me to Canberra to plead in the halls of Parliament House and dragged me out of bed to prepare for countless meetings and phone calls. Evenings were the same: kids to bed, Dad to the phone, the computer, the policy-writing, the discussion papers, and on it went. Maggie wore out the road between Nowra and Sydney.

Demanding as it was, this was a fabulous time from 2004 to 2007, where the pleasure of meeting other parents who experienced what we did led onto the next level of engagement—standing shoulder to shoulder with others to be the force for change. No more wishing for something better for our children, with these people we believed we could forge a safer, happier future. We all wanted to cure or prevent the diseases crippling our children, and to support as many families as possible.

The feeling that a great leap forward was tantalisingly close had a seductive power. So we just kept working at it. Midnight was an early night for months at a time.

The vehicle to our common goal was the successful formation of the unified national body. By July 2007 we had the outline of HeartKids Australia in place. We recruited a determined and resilient man, Neil McWhannell, to the role of CEO, introducing him to the dedicated network from all over Australia at the national conference, held in Adelaide.

Tremendous excitement attended the bringing together of the movers and shakers within the HeartKids movement to Adelaide that year. Decades of optimistic hope and struggle, balanced against fear and neglect, were concentrated into this one function at this singular point in time.

As chair, I felt an overwhelming responsibility to manage all the competing pressures of risk and opportunity. Despite all the time and effort we and many others had poured into the cause I feared eleventh-hour derailment. Human nature being what it is there were struggles and rivalries between states and between individuals: those for change and those against. Each state group was in a very different stage in its evolution. The whole thing could implode.

To my great satisfaction, implosion was not the outcome. Goodwill and good management rose to the surface. There was a fabulous feeling of consensus and resolution over the few days we gathered. The facilitator, Stephen Shepherd, was an old friend of mine. He brought such an acute mind and flawless diplomacy to his task that he would go on to become a unanimous choice to succeed me as chair. Our new CEO hit the ground running.

Having nursed so many aspects of the conference from conception to this safe delivery, I went for a drink with Maggie and a couple of other reforming allies. The success of the past several years of groundwork was ripe for the celebrating. As we charged our glasses, I burst into tears. My unexpected flood of distress stopped the conversation dead. As my companions consoled me, I was embarrassed and completely blindsided. Nothing in the years of activism and struggle had brought me close to tears. Now this!

I hadn't been self-aware enough to realise how invested I was in that event. My catharsis was safe to enjoy, sharing the table as I did with others who had also sacrificed, with their eyes on the same prize: a safer future for our children.

21

MAX MARTLY

There's something going on at this school.

— Max Martly

Make-A-Wish Australia did find a way to bring Malachy's wish to life. After months without word, Max confirmed the recruitment of a suitable and willing producer/director, leading to the arrival of Adrian Maher on the 'Life of Malachy' stage. Adrian brought know-how, energy and care to the task of making Malachy's writings screen-ready. Script drafts and edits went back and forth as I tried to temper Malachy's demand for absolute control of the project. Regrettably, I pushed some little amendments past Malachy, without staying fully true to his vision, distracted as I was by the competing demands of work and family. In much the same way as the greatest of artists agonises over their creative imperfections which we scarcely regard, Malachy was bugged by the departures. He reminded me often that the final screenplay was not the true writer's cut. For better or worse Adrian and I had used our adult diplomatic sense to work the story for ready consumption by a wider audience, not yet initiated into Malachy's fantasy world.

Screenwriting, filming, producing and screening the movie *Max Martly and the Fantastic Group* would all happen in a blur of efficient scheduling through the second half of 2007, fitted around a renovation of the family home.

Acknowledging then that any imperfections were the fault of myself and Adrian, a very satisfactory screenplay saw the Make-A-Wish movie entourage descend upon Nowra through the October school holiday period that year.

Malachy had long been friends with two identical twin sisters who were bright, energetic, and frequently part of our family social life, being the children of close friends. They shared with Malachy that keen-mindedness that bypassed social reticence— just friends without judgement. While their childhood friendships bounded along in platonic innocence, rumour had it one of the girls, Audrey, had once shared a kiss with Malachy at a Christmas party. Perhaps a subterranean frisson lingered, for when Malachy turned his attention to casting, sure enough his designated leading lady was Audrey. Malachy was a perfectionist, and I knew from our discussions he thought Audrey to be the most intelligent of his peers. Only the best and most trusted performers would be placed into the key roles in *Max Martly and the Fantastic Group*.

Integral to Malachy's vision for the film was his inclusion of his friends and family in the cast. He invested emotion in trying to balance people's talents and attributes with the prominence they had earned through loyal friendship or genetic bond. Close friends, like Ryan, naturally became the nucleus of the 'Fantastic Group', which also found space for Niamh and Seamus, size differences notwithstanding. Setting much of the action within a school, meant age range could be accommodated, with Imogen being both sister and senior student. The role of her classmates made room in the cast for friends of Imogen, including Malachy's particular buddy, Callum. Typecasting as parents was all it took to launch Maggie and me on the shared path to stardom.

Malachy's closest friend, Ryan, was typecast as his best mate. Ryan had been faultlessly loyal to Malachy from the first time they played together, willingly sharing the playground isolation dictated by Malachy's physical impairment. They had gone through kindergarten together, holidayed together, even been bullied together, and their friendship stayed unchanged, as it would for many years to come. For these boys, playing central roles in the *Max Martly* film together may well have been the origin of their enduring love of film as an artistic medium. The two friends would go on to spend much of their spare time as teenagers putting ideas out in the world, uploading their own film skits to the internet.

Guided by Adrian, and with his girlfriend helping marshal the troops, a tremendous feat of teamwork was extracted from Make-A-Wish staff and volunteers, the HeartKids CEO, friends and family.

Venues needed to execute the storyline were easily obtained. St Michael's Parish School graciously allowed us access to the buildings through the holiday period. This was particularly salient as the plot featured all manner of nefarious activities occurring on a school campus.

Malachy had a fold-out chair with a sign declaring its occupant to be DIRECTOR, and direct he did. The dance of creative urge with practical challenges and carrying the team along with the project ebbed and flowed, with Adrian doing a delightful job of making it work while ensuring Malachy's input was given prominence and his ownership of the project honoured. Eight-year-old Malachy brought such earnestness to the endeavour that he commanded respect from all of us. There was no shirking, no outsourcing of responsibility for the creative impetus. My film, my way.

Many lives have short periods that distinguish themselves from the sameness of passing time on either side. Bob Dylan sang of 'music in the cafés at night and revolution in the air', evoking a sense of purposeful existence, a time with meaning that would reach beyond the present. Something of that feeling attached to the filming of *Max Martly*. Each family involved in this grand cooperative work had briefing notes, schedules, instructions when to be where, in which outfit. So many small contributions flowed in bearing out the love and regard Malachy engendered. So many people gathered, unknowingly touched by the inclusive vision this little guy had, to fit us all into his chosen event.

As the pieces came together, we each had the chance to wrestle our own insecurities about our screen presence, or acting ability, to balance our scene-stealing urges against our theatrical limitations. Long stretches in the sun trying not to muff our lines or make them acceptably convincing, and repeated rejigging of sequences of action and dialogue, all conspired to establish this as a window outside the humdrum of ordinary living. It didn't matter so much what we did, as long as we were there for the ride.

Our household buzzed for days while guests came and went to the set and to our home, and we ticked off one scene after another. Malachy was central to most of the action so had the tightest of filming schedules, but there was no shortage of fun to go around for the bit players. Close scrutiny of the film will even show that one of our stars was taken ill during the shoot, but by a stroke of luck had an identical replacement in the wings.

The end product merely hints at the bonding that suffused this project, but on the ground I could feel the spirit building, a spark of life breathed into our band of child amateurs and their guardians. An unlikely common goal drew into sight as take followed take. It dawned on us that our lead man had given us all an experience to bank in wait for the next revolutionary period.

While it isn't the concluding scene of the movie itself, the last scene to be filmed involved mass participation as a band of students, led by the indefatigable Max Martly, uncovered the evil mystery afoot, rescuing two previously respectable teachers from the hypnotic spell of the plotting villain. In a triumphant scene the innocent parties wrestled them to the ground, disarming the teachers, casting their weapons onto the dirt, stamping them to pieces with alacrity.

'CUT, and WE ARE DONE!' cried Adrian.

We whooped and celebrated like mad things.

22

MAX AT THE ROXY

The red carpet is a beautiful situation for people. I think every-body appreciates it and loves it and honours it. Nobody really acts a fool because they know this is a one-time thing.

— Snoop Dogg

When *Max Martly and the Fantastic Group* premiered at Nowra's charmingly old-time picture theatre, the Roxy Cinema, nothing was held back. There was no place here for self-deprecatory reserve. The orders of the day were limousines, red carpet, fanfare and star power.

The child stars had a surprise to start their day. Their Premiere Gala experience began with the elegance, shining white pomp and tinted windows of a stretch limousine pulling up to the kerb outside our home. The icebox brimmed with cool drinks and treats. Plush carpet and the soothing chill of air conditioning welcomed Malachy and the others into the celebrity fold. The drive to the Roxy may be short but was luxurious to a degree befitting the occasion. A home-grown hero was bringing his first movie onto the silver screen of his waking dreams.

I didn't ride in the limousine, being well beyond the upper qualifying age limit for child stars, and neither was I 'in' on the organisation of the day, being in the unfamiliar role of charitable beneficiary. Make-A-Wish touchingly included our whole family as targets for the roll-out of Malachy's wish in its final realisation.

While the limo took a tour of local sights en route to the Roxy, Maggie and I made our own way there, in the process seeing what was in store for the gang of newly minted celebrities. A teeming throng of humanity, bustling with enthusiasm filled the street outside the cinema. The footpath was crowded beyond recognition, but for a cleared strip which would mark the course Malachy would follow from car to theatre.

The limo slid into place, the chauffeur drew open the door, and Malachy's foot reached across the kerb, resting in chuffed recognition on the deep red carpet installed for this moment. He stood to the cheers of the crowd, bubbling over in communal love and support for the beautiful boy and his inspiring wrestle with such a heavy weight of adversity. The collected goodwill of people from so many threads of the web of Malachy's life had found an avenue for expression. These were unforgettable, champagne moments in a life where each milestone was already laden with meaning beyond the ordinary.

Adjusting to the shock of such an uproarious welcome, Malachy and the others then observed the hush of the gathering. The resplendent source from which the hush descended wore such finery as to further mark the occasion as existing on a less real plane—complete with staff, waistcoat, and tails of scarlet fit to serve in the Queen's guard, was none other than the town crier. His bell rang out across the gathering, stilling the audience to receive announcement of the arrival of Malachy, and explain the occasion of this special premiere event. The crowd parted to allow passage of the honoured children. Dark glasses and conspiratorial glances intact, they strode the crimson pathway to the entrance of the Roxy, then up the stairs they climbed and into the complex.

Pragmatic survival of a small-town cinema into today's movie marketplace had long since demanded that the old-style massive cinema playing to a full house twice a year for Disney's latest, had given way to partitioning into several separate auditoria with fewer seats and smaller screens. Given the drawing power of *Max Martly and the Fantastic Group* the ticketholders had to make use of not one, but two of the cinemas. Nonetheless there was a necessary process of introduction and expressions of gratitude to undertake. For this, all the attendees crowded into one of the rooms, straining the capacity of both the space and the cooling system. Easing the responsibilities of stardom for Malachy, Seamus and Niamh had volunteered to speak on behalf of our family. Seamus was by now 12 and Niamh ten. Their balance of excitement and composure under the whisperings and scrutiny of the crowd squeezing in, flooded me with a warm satisfaction. That these little people were special and made more so by their entanglement in the care and love of their brother, was a clear, resounding subtext to their contribution. The two of them stood among the audience, cute beyond description, beaming with delight, oblivious to the nervousness that so often attends efforts at public speaking. The love and closeness between the children meant they all shared the glow of a bright, shiny beacon of survival against the odds, triumph over challenge, happiness in the face of gloom. Every mind in that room had pause to focus on all the good they desired for these innocents and their family. Such care could carry a family to the sky and back.

If only you could bottle that for use in the tougher times to follow.

The movie itself followed, warts and all, dare I say it! We watched as Max Martly uncovered a devious plot within the school aimed at nothing less than world domination, with an innocent misunderstood creature bearing the blame for countless wrongs along the way while a group of children pursued the truth, despite official obstruction and disregard. Along the way people got to move with the storyline, laugh at the actors, marvel at the ambitious production, and enjoy their own local sights and some familiar faces lighting up the screen. The town, our friends and relatives, had a sweet entertainment around which to rally to the cause. As the curtains drew at the final denouement, more was in store.

Out in the lobby, the stars had been coerced into being available for their public. Tables were set up, with cards and posters for signing. This taste of fame would not, as it turns out, gloss over the responsibilities to fans! The fledgling autographs would have plenty of practice that day, and no doubt tucked away in shoeboxes around Nowra to this day are souvenirs bearing the signature of Malachy and his co-stars, perhaps to be stumbled upon in some unpredicted moment, inspiring reminiscence.

It was a lovely day for the whole community to celebrate and remember. One of Malachy's many gifts to all of us.

23

A ROAST IN IRELAND

Security is mostly a superstition. It does not exist in nature,
nor do the children of men as a whole experience it. Avoid-
ing danger is no safer in the long run than outright exposure.
Life is either a daring adventure, or nothing.

— Helen Keller

With HeartKids Australia up and running and its first conference out of the way, an old itch reared its head.

Maggie's pitch had been refined and the decks cleared.

'Darling, you know how you've done what you needed to for
HeartKids Australia?'

'Yes?' was my cautious reply. Maggie continued.

'And you know Malachy is pretty stable, and none of the kids
have big exams coming up?'

Now I was sensing an ambush. 'Yes?'

'And your work is going along nicely? Well ... I'm resigning
from my job at HeartKids, and ... we should move to Ireland. Siva
can take over your patients. We won't get a better chance, Dom. I
really think it's now or never.'

She was right. In support of Maggie's case, my most recent
registrar was an excellent doctor and keen to stay on in the practice.
The ready sensible excuses that had got me out of this escapade for
a number of years had all neatly evaporated within a few months
of each other.

119

The emotional case for Ireland was also fuelled by the eccentric small-town quirkiness of the TV show *Ballykissangel* and the scattered experiences we had of gregarious, funny, friendly Irish people in their travels Downunder.

It was time to test whether I truly believed adventure was more important to us than safety. Some capacity for reinvention was almost a matter of pride for us, having loved the places and people that taking chances had thrown our way in life.

By August, Maggie had won me over. I revisited my earlier homework on Irish locum agencies, and we made plans for a fresh adventure.

The year of 2007 was drawing to a close and excitement overrode nervous apprehension as we crammed our lives into one large suitcase each and one carry-on bag. No luxuries required. We were going to live lean and go with the flow. Malachy's cardiologist, Dr Cooper, gave us the name of a colleague in Dublin whom we could consult along the way, a doctor he regarded highly. We hoped against hope this wouldn't be needed, banking on this being the grandest of adventures.

Snow, though a rarity in Ireland, was on hand to greet us at Dublin Airport on a bitter January morning in 2008. The warm socks we'd acquired in anticipation of the hostile climate had helped Malachy's feet to sweat and swell enough to cause trouble during the flight over, then left him below par for the challenge of speeding out of the terminal in sleet and snow to meet the coach. Arriving in central Dublin, our full complement of luggage needed to be dragged through the rain-drenched streets to the Avalon House backpackers' hostel—a daunting physical challenge for the able-bodied, for Malachy, this was near impossible. Slowing to his speed was trying in any conditions, but at zero degrees, in rain, lost in a strange city on the other side of the world, it was exasperating. Some of our travelling party felt the need to express this exasperation, repeatedly, and then to increase the volume when the hostel presented a confronting parade of young backpackers in their y-fronts and an ensuite bathroom smelling of untreated sewage.

After a few days in Dublin, which included my orientation as a medical locum, we bundled into a hire car and drove ourselves south to County Waterford where, in theory, I would help start up a new urgent-care medical clinic.

While the cold was hard on Malachy, he made no complaints, approaching the Irish sojourn with enthusiasm, buoyed as he was by his recent success as a moviemaker. He enrolled in school, developed a taste for the Irish breakfast, never complete without both black and white pudding, and settled in to immerse himself in our new life. He and Seamus relished gathering samples of the local accents and mimicking them with fair accuracy. The stronger versions of the Waterford accent proved great fun and brought a different kind of music to the household. They babbled on together in their own world enhanced by enjoyment of the unfamiliar sounds and sights of Ireland's so-called Sunny South East. This label, the tourist brochures advised, is earned by virtue of the southeast region suffering 'precipitation on *only* 73% of days'.

Alien and isolated on our arrival in Eire, our new home was Bob's Lodge, a farmhouse in the local equivalent of the middle of nowhere. My work life became marooned on the rocks of Irish organisational chaos and petty local conflict. The clinic I'd been employed to manage would not open until eight months after our arrival, and the local doctors were at loggerheads with the locum agency that had brought me to their door. The bleak and bitter weather seemed at times to dictate the mood of the locals who, with a few exceptions, were slow to welcome us intruders.

Ireland's history was that of a mass exporter of humans. Clearly the import business would take some adjusting to.

Being cast as the visiting locum, the protection of my status as boss of my own dominion which I'd enjoyed since 1996, was stripped away. Apparently, we locums were a very lowly species on the medical pecking order, useful only to fill whatever gaps the locals found inconvenient. My locum work found me in odd jobs all over Ireland. My varied tasks included visiting police cells at three in the morning, being stranded in a housing unit with a suicidal woman and her kitchen knife, tearing up the Cork Road to a four-car pile-up, sorting a catatonic student frozen on his feet, and preserving an ageing lord with his houseful of servants and Dobermans. At times I felt like a frightened first-year intern all over again.

But there we were in Ireland. Adventure has a price!

Malachy, too, was outside his comfort zone, confronting the cold at every turn, and with the social lie of the land slow to reveal itself. In the early months it was dark when he left for school, and again when he returned home.

All the children found themselves thrust into an extremely insular life. We fell for the romance of living way out of town down a narrow moss-lined road. The quaintly named Bob's Lodge was a typical, sparely designed Irish country house, with a grey, box-like two-storey structure, narrow windows evenly spaced across front and back. There were very few close neighbours, and only Niamh had someone her age to play with. There was really nowhere for the children to escape the constant attention of their parents, and conversely, we were granted the chance to observe them far more keenly than we ever could at home.

Diversions were badly needed. One discovery that helped inject some fun into the stillness of remote country life was a recreational business called 'Laser Blast' in a nearby coastal town. Laser Blast involved a battle game, fought in teams, inside a warehouse. Each player carried a laser gun and wore a harness with targets front and back. A player would score points by hitting the targets on any member of the opposing team, who would then be disabled for several seconds, allowing time to escape before they could either shoot or be shot once more. It was brilliant for Malachy, because he had a team that could cover for him when tired, he could hide when needing a breather, and you could easily cut him some slack once he'd worn a shot. Trained by years of appropriate accommodation, it was simple for us to give leeway to Malachy, leave him space to gasp his way back into shape as required, and finish a session with smiles all round.

As friendships grew at school, one of Malachy's classmates held a birthday party, choosing Laser Blast as the venue for the celebration. Familiar as we were with the game and the set-up, we were excited that this was a party purpose-built for our boy. We dropped him off and the games began. The boys geared up and divided into red and blue teams in the usual fashion and sprung off into the game. Mac was in his element, knowing the game and loving the camaraderie. He wandered the obstacles, shooting and ducking with the rhythm of a master spy, then of course, was forced by his infirmity to pause to regain his breath. An enemy approached in the form of his best new schoolmate, Ruairi (Rory), who was sharp enough to shoot first, leaving Malachy to take his breather. As the armour rebooted, just before Malachy had firepower, 'Bing Bing', he was shot again. Ruairi had waited nearby for Mac to reboot. Several seconds passed, 'Bing Bing' again. Easy points on offer here. Seconds again, as Malachy still heaved with breathlessness, unable to run away, 'Bing Bing'.

'Ruairi' he pleaded, 'go and shoot someone else. I can't run.'

'Bing, Bing' came the answer, as the Heart Kid was forced to remain missing in action, powered down by his friend.

'Please, Ruairi!'

Malachy by this age was somewhere near average height, but still painfully thin, and relatively weak as a result of his limited exertion. He, nonetheless, had a normal level of feistiness. Despite the caution we urged, he was unafraid to give someone a serve, though generally more inclined to negotiate his way through troubles. On this occasion he took the route of negotiation, though some urgency was desired given the competitive nature of the game.

Further pleading with his assailant didn't gain the accustomed fair go for Malachy, who lost his cool, grabbing Ruairi at the neck, pushing him against the wall, and pleading, 'Go and shoot some-one else'.

Maggie was called to collect Malachy who, it was reported, had viciously attacked the poor child, in a mean act for which he would be made to serve penance.

It was heartbreaking for us to see our son, the outsider, apparently dash the best friendship he had going, in an act of anger. More so for Malachy, from whose perspective his best friend had just single-handedly ruined the most fun he'd had all year, repeatedly refusing to let him into the game. He raged about the betrayal as we sought to eke out the story of what had happened and form our judgement of the event.

The following Monday, with resumption of school, Malachy unprompted sought out his nemesis to apologise. Whatever resentment he bore he dispensed with. Pride was swallowed and reconciliation addressed. That afternoon at school pick-up, Malachy sought out the mother of the protagonist, explaining to her his sorrow for what had happened and his wish to make it up to Ruairi. An invitation to our house was offered. A children's misunderstanding was to be readily patched over by the children themselves. Justice in action! The response from the mother: 'No, Malachy. It's too soon for that, too soon for Ruairi to forgive.' The adult had spoken. True to her word, forgiveness was not to be found in that quarter.

A highlight of the Grade Two calendar in Irish schooling was the celebration of First Holy Communion, still at that time a full 'Brides of Christ' experience, with white dresses and veils for the girls, full school uniform, complete with long-sleeved shirts, grey suit pants and a tie for the boys. Parties in honour of the event were weeks in the preparation. Some of the girls would have fittings as if for a wedding dress, which would feature in the family albums for time immemorial. Malachy's school, a boys-only school in a tiny seaside village, shared the occasion with the local girls' school, adding the excitement of meeting the girls to the pomp and austerity of the occasion. Thankfully, Malachy's ostracism following the incident at Laser Blast was fading in intensity by Communion time. It was a surprise then, to arrive and find that our son was the only one dressed in keeping with the established rules of decorum and the advice from the school. The boys' mothers had phoned around and agreed that, since it was a small year, and we're all friends here, we needn't knock ourselves out with all the trouble of fancy dress. So, everyone was called, and the rules were shifted. Everyone but Malachy. One child was starched and dressed to the nines, the others were as they pleased.

Not a whisper of apology did we hear for this attempt at isolation of our child. Nor did we hear a whisper of upset from the victim himself, whose ability saw him appointed as a reader for the liturgy. This job he performed with clear diction, even pacing and loud projection. A model of equanimity, Malachy didn't waste a split second on distress over his exclusion from the group, and regardless of any machinations, mixed happily with the congregation.

'Good man, yourself,' as they say in Waterford.

As much as I may have been tempted to resent this intrusion of belligerent adult pettiness into the innocent world of the nine-year-old child, Malachy's gracious persistence in ignoring the ill spirit of it won out over any concerns. Cheerfulness was innate to Mac, who was loved without judgement by his brother and sisters and displayed a tremendous capacity to withhold judgment from others. Barely midway through childhood, he knew from somewhere to see conflict from the perspective of the other.

Busy trying to teach, here I was learning at the feet of my child.

The year in our ancestral home presented many highlights, uplifting moments and heartwarming experiences alongside the struggles against loneliness and the elements. Not least among the pleasures was the friendship we developed with the neighbours across the street, who went to lengths to welcome and support us, and whose children shared friendship with ours, especially Niamh who shared countless hours across the lane with her classmate.

We used to love seeing the children working their way up the small hill from the bus stop at the bottom of the lane. Memorably on one occasion as spring passed into summer, the Irish children struggled up the hill, as breathless as Malachy, beads of sweat erupting on their lips and foreheads, as their cheeks flushed red in the heat, while our two, accustomed to warmer climes remained cool and dry. 'You look hot, children!' cried Maggie. 'Ooh, Maggie, it's ROASTING!' complained the sweaty, red-faced locals. The thermometer read 16 degrees Celsius. The Irish idea of what constitutes 'Roasting' is a family in-joke to this day, roasting as we do through much of the Australian winter.

By May, some warmth crept onto the thermometers of Ireland's South East, and our thoughts turned to one of our primary aspirations for this sojourn in the northern hemisphere: European travel. From Ireland, a stone's throw and 50 Euros was all it took to see us herded onto a Ryanair flight and on our way to Majorca.

The flight to France and on to Spain happily coincided with the first warm days of the year; we loved that near-forgotten feeling of the sun warming through your skin. Warmth into your bones was rediscovered the day we landed on Majorca, as the mercury climbed to 40 degrees, somewhat more like what we called ROASTING! It was a heavenly feeling of homecoming. I hardly realised how difficult I found the cold until that moment of bliss in the dry heat of Palma de Majorca.

It does no justice to the wonderful people we met, the culture we imbibed, or the fabulous experiences we shared in Ireland, but it was no surprise on returning home to hear my children's response when asked, 'What was the best thing about Ireland?'

Unscripted, to a person, their response: 'Majorca!'

24

TRAVELS WITHIN TRAVELS

Dwell on the beauty of life. Watch the stars, and see yourself running with them.

— Marcus Aurelius

By day two or three in Majorca we were once more used to the burning heat, and deep familiar warmth of the sun. It was like a little bit of Australia in the Mediterranean Sea. Free expressions of glee and excitement filled the air in a way the cold cloistered wetness of Ireland seemed to prohibit. Growing up in the 'Great South Land', warmth and freedom seem natural bedfellows. Climbing my way up the ladders of a giant waterslide in Majorca I could hardly conceive how Franco's dictatorial ways could have subdued the joyful spirit of this holiday mecca. The delighted squeals of children and the whoops of adults mingled high above the water as I climbed further, my legs trembling with fatigue and adrenaline-tinged fear. The sun belted down on my skin, making the plunge to the water below all the more enticing.

Seamus and Imogen were with me, both up for the challenge of the huge drop, though content for Dad to bite the bullet first. A loud repeated crackling noise that at first had seemed mechanical in origin proved to be produced by the belting of speeding bodies against the trickle of water lubricating the monster slide. From the top, on the cusp of the drop-off, the slide looked higher than I had anticipated.

Meanwhile down below a more modest feat was proving challenging to a nine-year-old boy with congenital heart disease.

Malachy had never mastered swimming. His heart seemed to find the pressure changes and continued exertion too much, too quickly. On the face of it a waterslide did away with this problem, as gravity would power the child through the water without the need for exertion. But then one had to land, usually plunging into a pool at the bottom of the ride, before swimming to the safety of the exit. All was struggle at ground level, as Maggie tried to find a slide that would start with a climb Malachy could manage, provide a ride he would enjoy, then deliver him to a pool in which he would not drown. She stumbled on a pair of slides that suited, with a short climb she could help Mac with, and a shallow enough dumping pool she could wade into, as rescuer, at the finish.

I bucked myself up for a task my experience told me would be tough, but rewarding, while Malachy had to wrestle the limits of his ability merely to have a passably good time. It was something of a mirror to our experience of Ireland. Nothing in our year to date had been as easy as it had appeared in anticipation. By the time we embarked on the trip to Majorca, Mac and I were both in need of some restoration. Western Water Park, Majorca, was playing its part.

Atop the highest ladder at the park, the urge to freeze ran fleetingly up my spine. The young attendant had seen this countless times before and cared not for my pause and preparatory breath. He hustled. I plunged.

The safety of the platform fell away, and I scorched down the slide, gaining speed as the parting water crackled against my skin and flew off into the air above. Gravity pushed harder as I reached the lower slope, where the near vertical grade levelled out, and smacked into the shallow fluid level of still water at the base of the slide. Such pain! Such pleasure! The exhilarating rush blasted away the cobwebs of pent-up frustration. Seamus and Imogen came thundering down behind me, equally thrilled, equally keen to head back up for another blast.

Niamh and Maggie, meanwhile, had seen Malachy enjoy his first momentum-driven shot down his own version of the giant slide. Niamh waited at the bottom to plunge in and catch the non-swimmer as he emerged. The emergence came, as we had hoped against hope, with a beaming smile. His first taste of the speed of a waterslide was to his liking, as was the second, the third, and so on. What relief and joy.

Majorca would offer other delightful experiences, including paella by the waterfront, the balmy warmth of the Mediterranean Sea, and the irresistible charm of majestic olive trees and grand old buildings, older than the official life of the Australian nation.

A re-set had occurred by the time we were back on damp Irish soil. We would continue to be challenged in various ways, not least the near exhaustion of our savings, but nothing so difficult as to damage our guiding belief that adventure beats safety. After all, who can predict when a bank of joyful experience may need to be drawn on as a buffer against boredom or the assault of tragic events?

Highlights of Malachy's adventures beyond Ireland that year would include visits to Paris and London, to Windsor Castle, Bath and Oxford. In Bath we would be guided by our English host for the week, Rachael, a penfriend I had established when I was 12, but until then never met. Malachy would travel through Wales and fly to Germany. We would pile into a mobile home in Germany and use it to explore Belgium and the Netherlands, and to see the terraced gardens of Luxembourg. Malachy would ascend the Eiffel Tower with his family, visit one of Disney's theme parks and be photographed eating snail.

One of our stops on the road in Germany was the picturesque Heidelberg, where we set up camp on the river with our six-berth vehicle. Though it was barely past July the children were pleased to discover a Christmas store in the centre of this historic city. None of us had experienced Europe at Christmas, so we weren't prepared for the bounty behind that quaint decorative shopfront.

Entering the shop, a melodic bell was triggered by the swing of the door and, as the children looked ahead, their eyes widened. Unexpectedly there were multiple stories in a vaulted expanse, where every inch of floor and shelf was crowded to overflowing with handcrafted goods. So beautiful were all the toys and decorations, the children hardly knew where to look, every glance demanded exclamations of pleasure or surprise. From tiny to huge and all sizes between, it seemed Santa's elves had a summer getaway. Imogen and Niamh declared immediately their intent never to leave the store, and I must confess I'd happily have lost a day in there myself. Every imaginable simply engineered wonder, and some complex ones as well, were crafted to perfection and spread on the shelves for our perusal. A three-inch Santa Claus, who climbed swiftly up a pair of ropes, gently tugged by the fascinated Niamh, found its way into her possession. To this day he repeats his merry climb in our hall every Christmas.

Malachy humoured his old Dad in the town of Trier, famous for its Roman era Porta Nigra (Black Gate) and other ruins less well-preserved, by taking an active interest in the birthplace of the man we jokingly referred to as 'Uncle Karl'. This was in reference to my leftward political leanings. Karl Marx was born in Trier in 1818, and his original home is preserved as a museum. Malachy was fascinated by the way one man's ideas could so influence people more than a hundred years beyond his death, or so he said! At this point in our travels Mac had taken to wearing a bandanna in the German national colours. To my mind, as Malachy parked himself on the kerb outside 'Uncle Karl's House', that bandanna subliminally reinforced Malachy's social justice warrior credentials. Its black, red and yellow striping matched the colours of the flag of Aboriginal Australia. The bandanna conveyed a casual disregard for accepted fashions and pointed to emerging coolness in the young Heart Kid from Nowra.

Stitch-by-stitch, every experience wove something more into Malachy's personality. Every collected memory might yet serve as the template for a new idea. I don't know if it was born of his own trauma or tinged with prescience, or just inherent to his nature, but Malachy was forever interested in things. He had a hunger to experience and to understand.

25

SOUNDTRACK OF THE PRIMARY YEARS

It will not be a surprise to you to learn I'm more interested in the future of the Arctic Circle than the future of the Arctic Monkeys.

— Gordon Brown

Sharing music within the family, discovering different tastes in keeping with each personality, and pondering what, if any meaning this carried, was a background hobby that brought mutual pleasure in the family. There would usually be some music playing in the background at home, and often discussion about the qualities of the bands or genres. One of my great pleasures with the process of negotiating the choice of music in the more focused sound environment of the car, where we spent a lot of time together.

Music for the road was an ever-changing smorgasbord, somehow different from music for home. I still love that feeling as the road opens up and a tune kicks in. It doesn't matter a whole lot what it is: sentimental anthems recalling trips of yesteryear, favourite songs for the mood of the moment, or the chance to blast and acquaint with something new and unfamiliar. When Maggie and I travelled around Australia before we started our family, our battle-weary Daihatsu Delta only contained a tape deck which was all we needed. In our minds we heard the opening chords of the next song even as the last was still playing out, each track waiting its turn in line, in order as ordained by the musician. We knew the music as albums, with a mood that ebbed and flowed through their course, this balance being an art form of its own. The opening stanza of any Tracy Chapman song still makes me feel I'm rushing across the Nullarbor with a diesel engine whirring away beneath the seat. The expanse that stretched out ahead of us included both the physical desert and the great unknowable life to come.

As our babies started to arrive, so too did the musical revolution that was the compact disc, with a false but alluring promise of scratch-proof indestructability, and a clarity of sound that would see them dispatch the much-loved cassette to history's scrapheap in the blink of an eye. When Malachy arrived we officially passed what we termed the 'Tarago Threshold'—the point at which your children no longer legally fit in a station wagon and you move up to a people carrier. This entailed acquisition of a CD-enabled car, just as the parents tired of The Wiggles and The Hooley Dooleys and started trying out what I thought of as 'real music' on the children. Featuring in the conversion were the Red Hot Chilli Peppers (with language editing), Ben Harper, The Oils, Nick Cave and later, some Jack Johnson and The Beautiful Girls. After alternating the 'real' and 'children's genres the former scored more hits than misses. The children started requesting our music in preference to theirs. Very discerning.

Malachy was compiling bunches of tunes before he could write or spell. To put the CD called *Mac's Rocn Celekshen* in the player now, immediately transports me back to the time of its making. The tunes we heard on high rotation through Mac's early school years have a power to recreate the mood of the time. It was a simple time for us when all we had to do was love our children unconditionally and dream of their futures.

Malachy's music taste was precocious. He seemed to have some themes, or unifying vibes, even as a six-year-old. He knew what he liked, which included humour, a meaningful edge to the lyrics, and a good guitar hook. Liam Lynch and Big Audio Dynamite got a run, Peter Garrett and Midnight Oil remained on their pedestal next to the White Stripes and the Chilli Peppers. The CD player was our best friend on our great Australian road trip in 2004. John Butler and Jack White probably ended up the ruling artists for that trip, alternating with Stephen Fry's reading of the *Harry Potter* series of books. The familiar chords of Butler's *Zebra* or *The White Stripes* or *Seven Nation Army* reliably send me back in time to that family odyssey.

In later years the arrival of the iPod put a dent in this particular style of family time our children, who had always been chatty and responsive during car trips, all of a sudden grew silent. Tiny white ear plugs were the visible hint as to why they were no longer responding to other humans. I was not content to let the social dimension of music die without a fight. For as long as we could Maggie and I enforced the rule that car trips were social time in which people would converse, and music would be played out loud, shared, with each of us taking a turn as DJ. In time people's tastes diverged so much that personal iPods became accepted for long trips, but the musical melting pot of those days remains a very fond memory.

Uprooting for Ireland included stripping back our possessions to a bare minimum. Our music collection was reduced to the beginnings of an iTunes library on the family laptop or suffer the offerings of Irish commercial radio. Australia's Triple J quickly became beloved in our recollection when we were forced to suffer its withdrawal. After a couple of months in Ireland we were feeling the pain as a handful of songs catchy enough, but not apparently meeting our deeper listening needs, dominated every radio station in the Emerald Isle.

This pain of longing for satisfactory music we could enjoy together eased a little around my birthday, after Maggie bought me two new CDs—one from The Foo Fighters, and more importantly, the Arctic Monkeys' *Favourite Worst Nightmare* which came to represent that year almost as much as anything did. The album has a raw, driving Indie sound, brimful of intense early career energy, typical of a band yet to prove itself. The children acquired an enthusiastic taste for the style of delivery, the content, and gradually the whole persona of the band. Seamus and Malachy would sing along with each other over and again, enjoying the cadence and complexity of the lyrics, and the retreat into their unshakeable bond of brotherhood. Isolated in our farmhouse, it felt as though the Arctic Monkeys were our secret undiscovered jewel of the music world. It still feels that way, even after sharing them with thousands of others in big music venues.

As we lived well out of town and our activities were spread widely, driving was a constant in Ireland, so we heard those two albums over and over. Without any grand moment to signify it, Malachy's primary musical allegiance shifted permanently, from Midnight Oil to the Arctic Monkeys.

Malachy dug up some gems amongst the Irish commercial radio music, with the common theme of Indie. We whiled away time with a splash of such indie darlings as The Kooks, The Fratellis, and The Killers. The Killers' prized lyric 'It's Indie rock and roll for me' would become something of an unspoken musical motto for Malachy in years to come.

Another type of music we would hear over and over that year, was the sound of Imogen on the piano, possibly the means by which she expressed her emotions. Minor keys suited the angst of a teenager adrift in a foreign land, remote from all familiar things and people. My feelings when I recall the lounge room in Bob's Lodge are irredeemably linked to the lilting sadness and uncertainty of a brief piece lifted from the *Corpse Bride* soundtrack, written by Danny Elfmann, famous for composing the theme tune for *Buffy the Vampire Slayer*. *Corpse Bride*'s forlorn hero, Walter, has fallen into unrequited love, and is proving fumblingly incapable of cementing the union. Walter sits at a grand piano to fill a haunted mansion with the beautiful sounds of an ode to his pained love.

A maudlin cry to the unattainable object of his desire. As the tune builds to a passionate crescendo his reverie clunks discordantly to a sudden close. He is interrupted... *SHE* is there. (Gulp) Many times that year I found myself in the process of being swept along by the aching, sad music, and forgetting myself, got snapped back to reality by the tune's abrupt conclusion. Fool me once...

The sharing of music in Ireland also included playing lots of guitar. Most days closed with me sitting in Niamh and Malachy's room, perched on either of their beds, strumming and singing lullaby snippets of Bob Dylan, Bob Marley, the Four Non Blondes and others until both sank into their dreams. I also had the chance to play a little with our neighbour, who participated in a music circle at a local pub—a tiny, thatched cottage on a country lane. It was here that we experienced the celebrated communal musicality of the Irish. Sad folk tunes of loss and infidelity abounded. On one memorable occasion, with a full house of traditional musicians taking turns to share one mournful tune after another, the woman next to me craned over to whisper, 'Thank Christ for this GFC— we'll finally get some new songs!'

Within our family music culture, 2008 was a period when a growing iTunes library rendered the CD obsolete. We were excited to discover that shopping to suit one's musical tastes could be undertaken with ease from any computer. This would prove a boon to Malachy. He and I found great pleasure whiling away some father-son time hunting, sampling, praising and dissing, learning the nuance of where music fitted in each other's perceptions.

We all came to recognise the qualities of his preferred sound, the 'Malachy Music' which would help define aspects of the man he became.

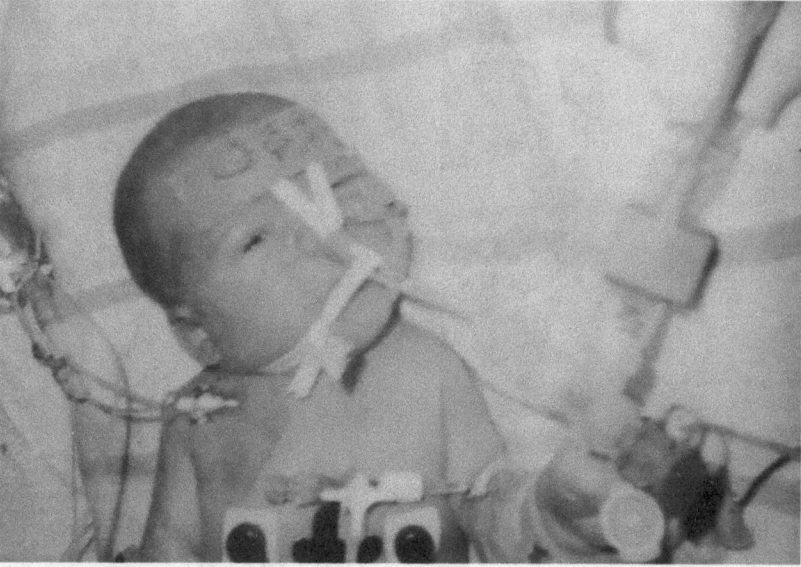
First eye contact with Malachy, snapped on 8th March in ICU, Children's Hospital, Randwick, Sydney.

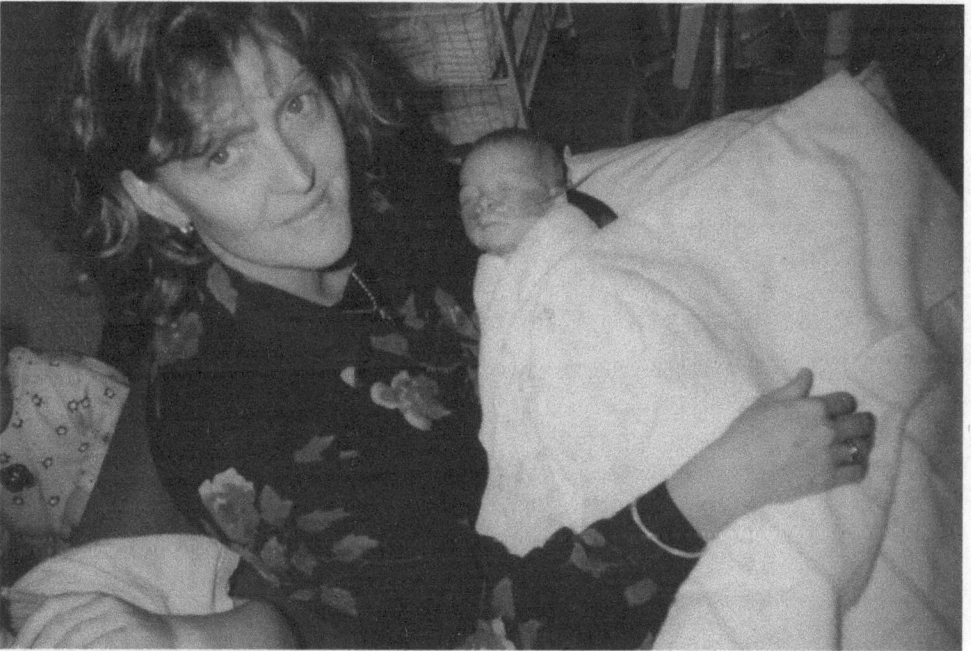
Maggie didn't get to hold baby Malachy for about 4 weeks.

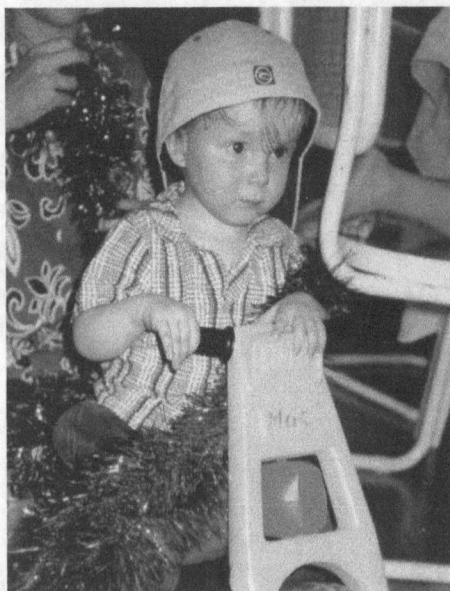

Two-year-old Malachy found his legs on a trike.

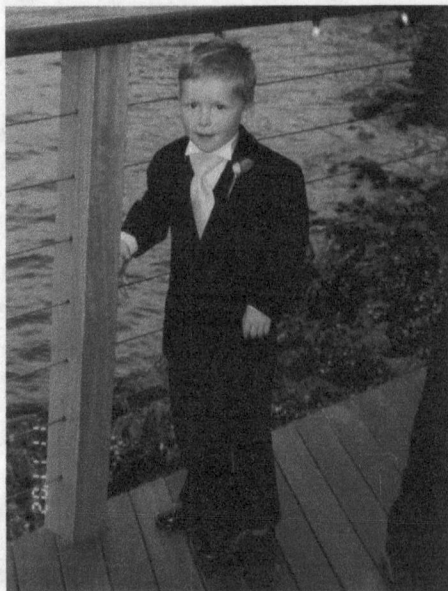

Malachy at his cousin's wedding, November 2002.

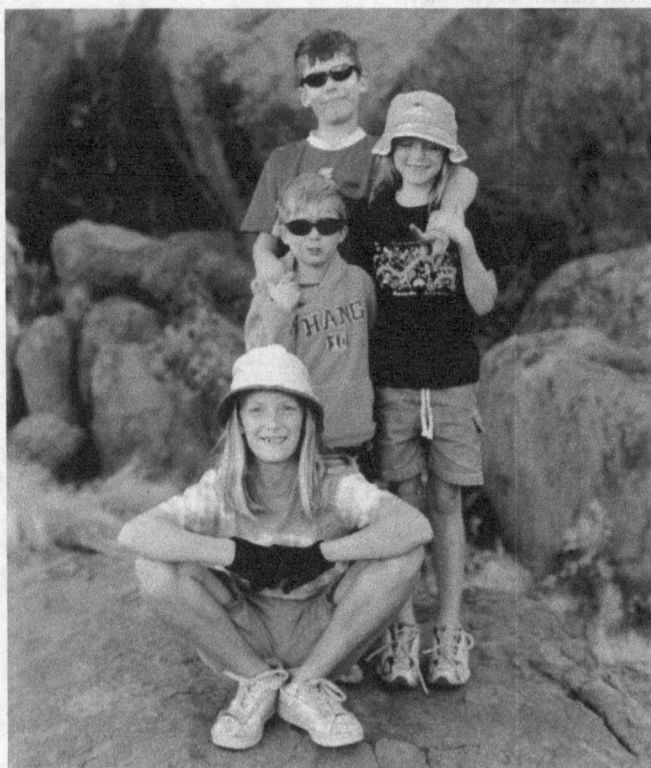

Playing it cool at Uluru, 2004.

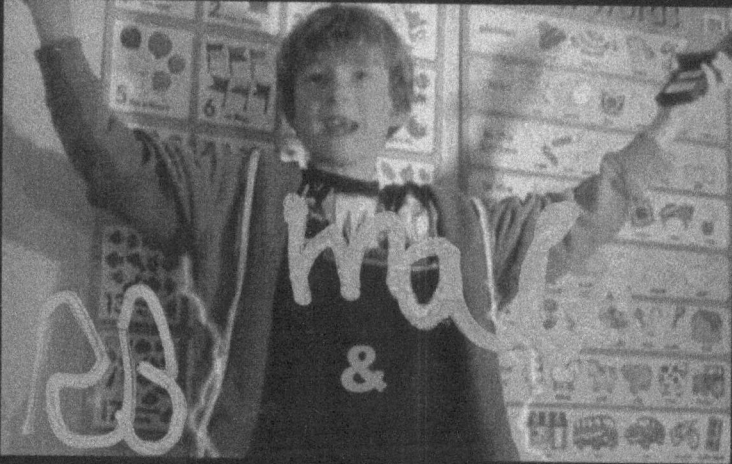
Malachy's autographed flyers for his Max Martly movie premiere, 2007.

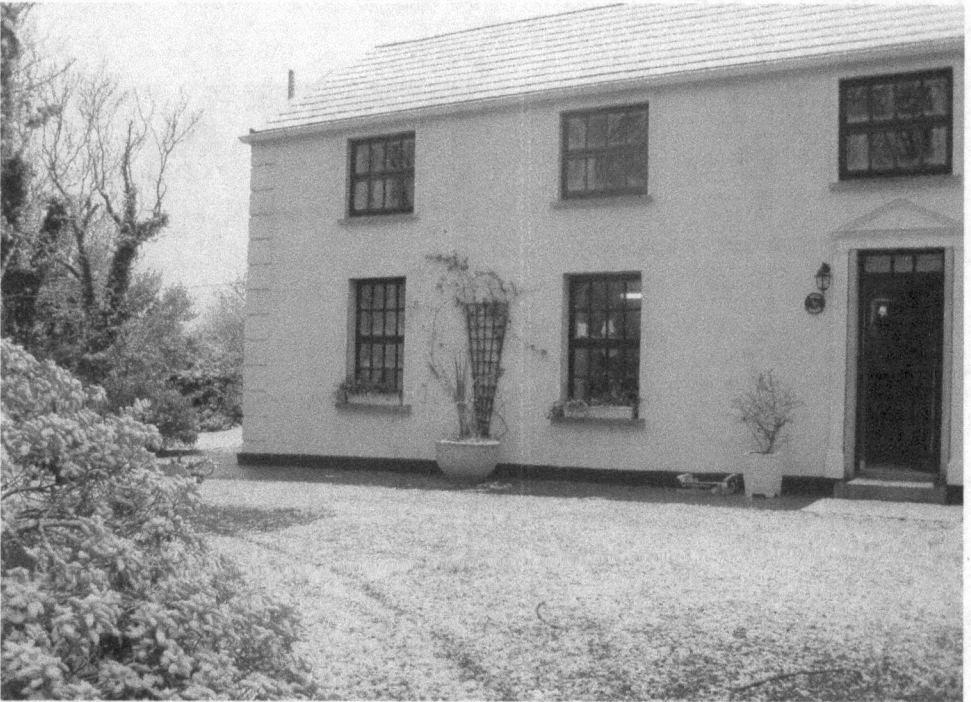
Home during 2008: Bob's Lodge in County Waterford, Ireland.

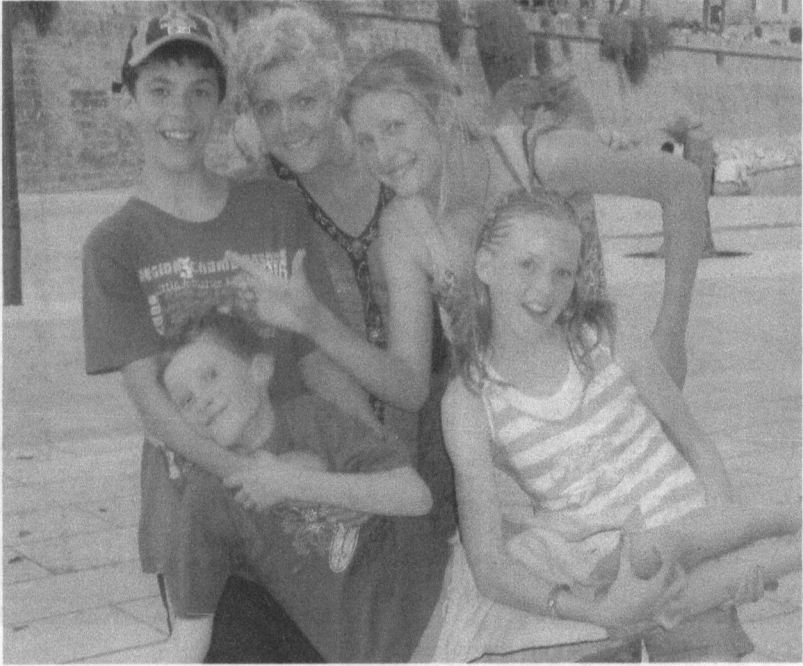

The family getting much-needed sunshine, Majorca, July 2008.

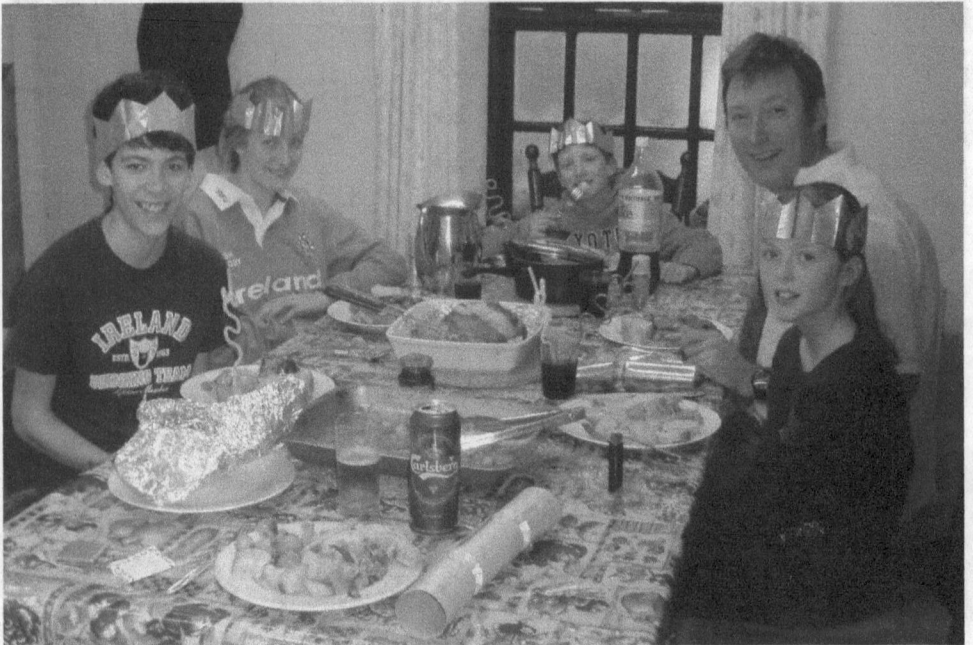

Maggie prepared a Christmas feast for the ages in Ireland.

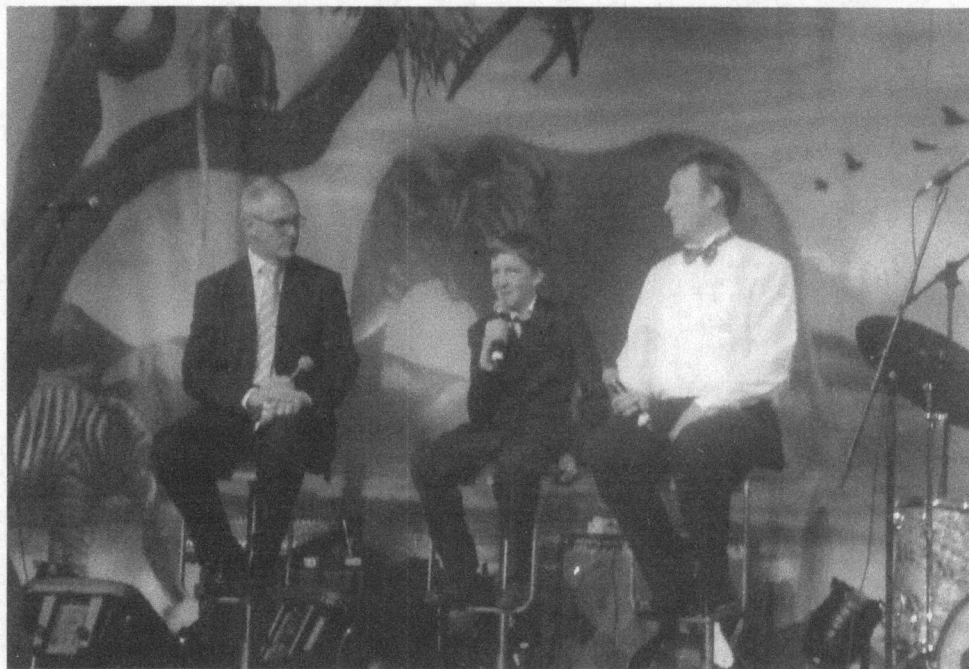
Malachy declaring himself 'proud of being blue' at the HeartKids NSW ball, September 2010.

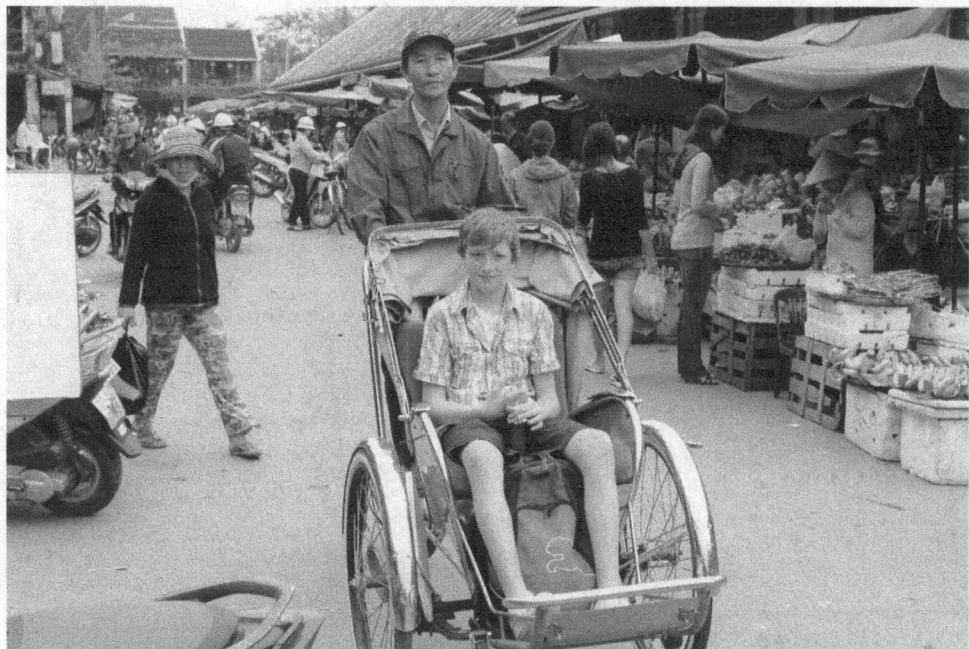
Malachy needed hauling in Vietnam, January 2012.

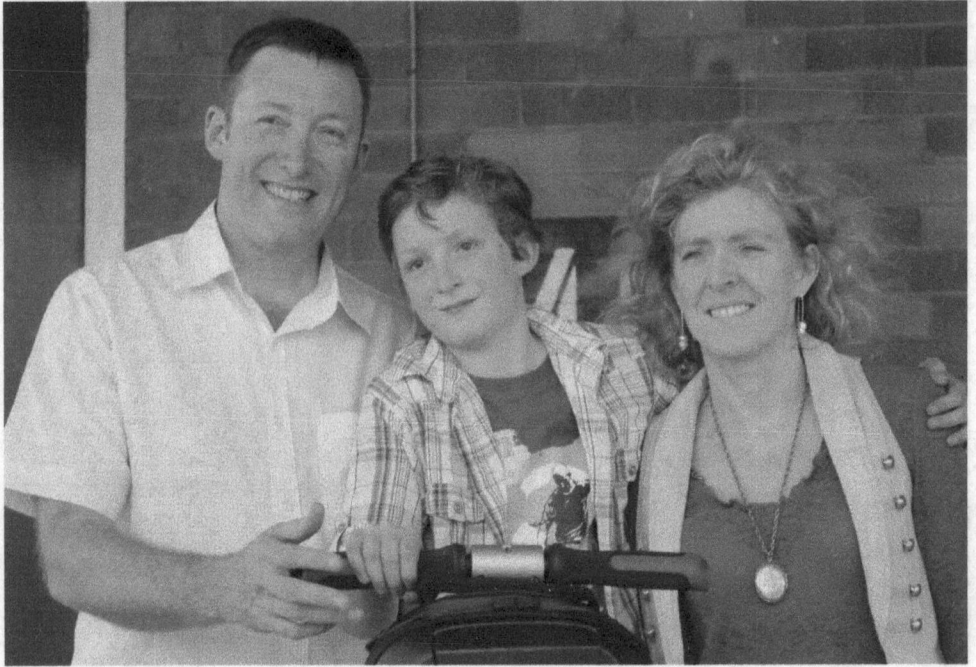

Dom, Maggie and Malachy claimed possession of the Segway, 2009.

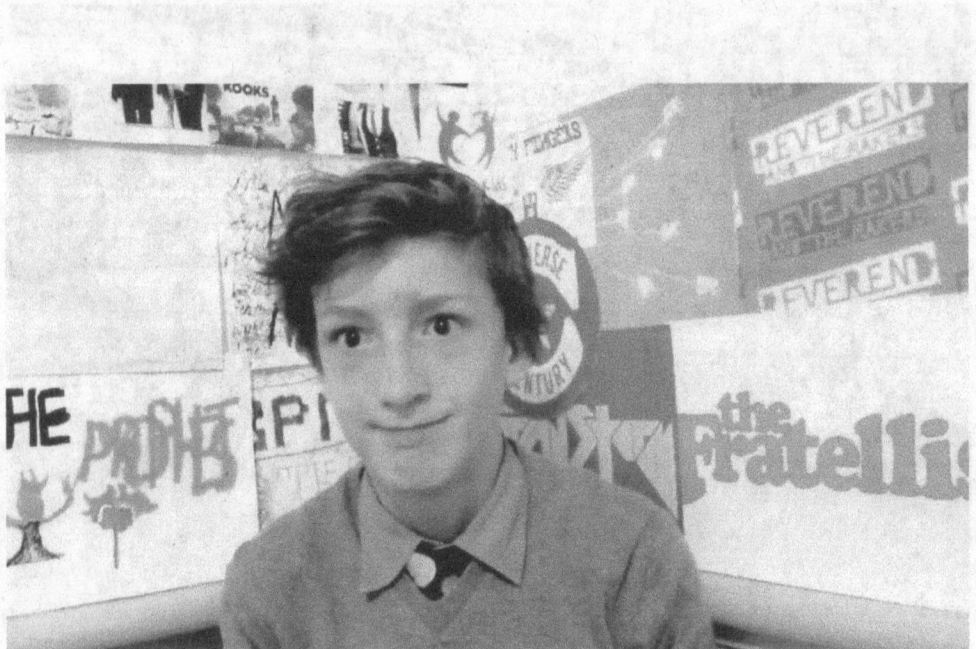

Malachy filmed for YouTube in his bedroom, framed by his 'wall of awesome'.

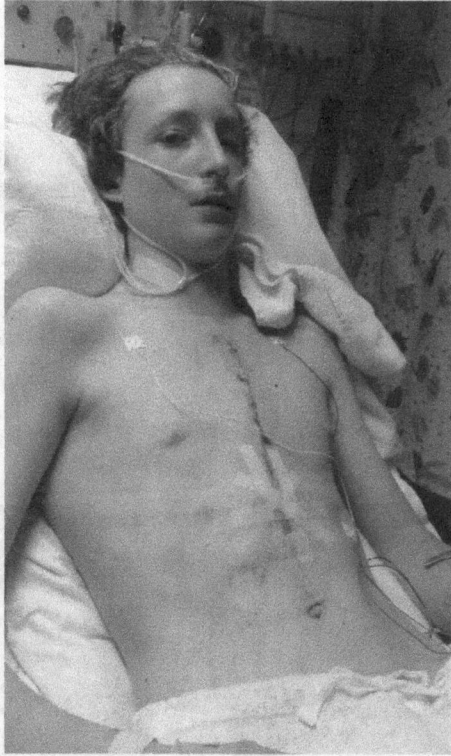

It was a tough recovery for Malachy at Westmead Children's Hospital, Sydney, around the Ides of March, 2013.

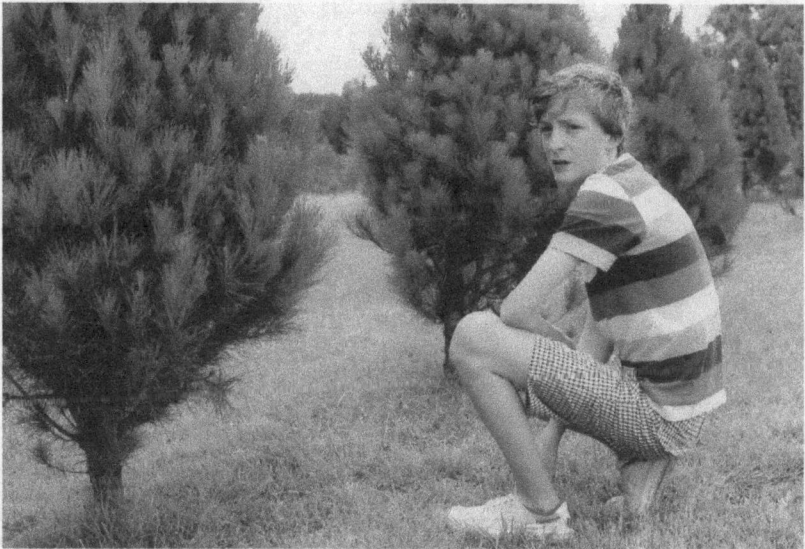

Malachy looking for a Christmas tree, nearly 14 years old, in December 2012.

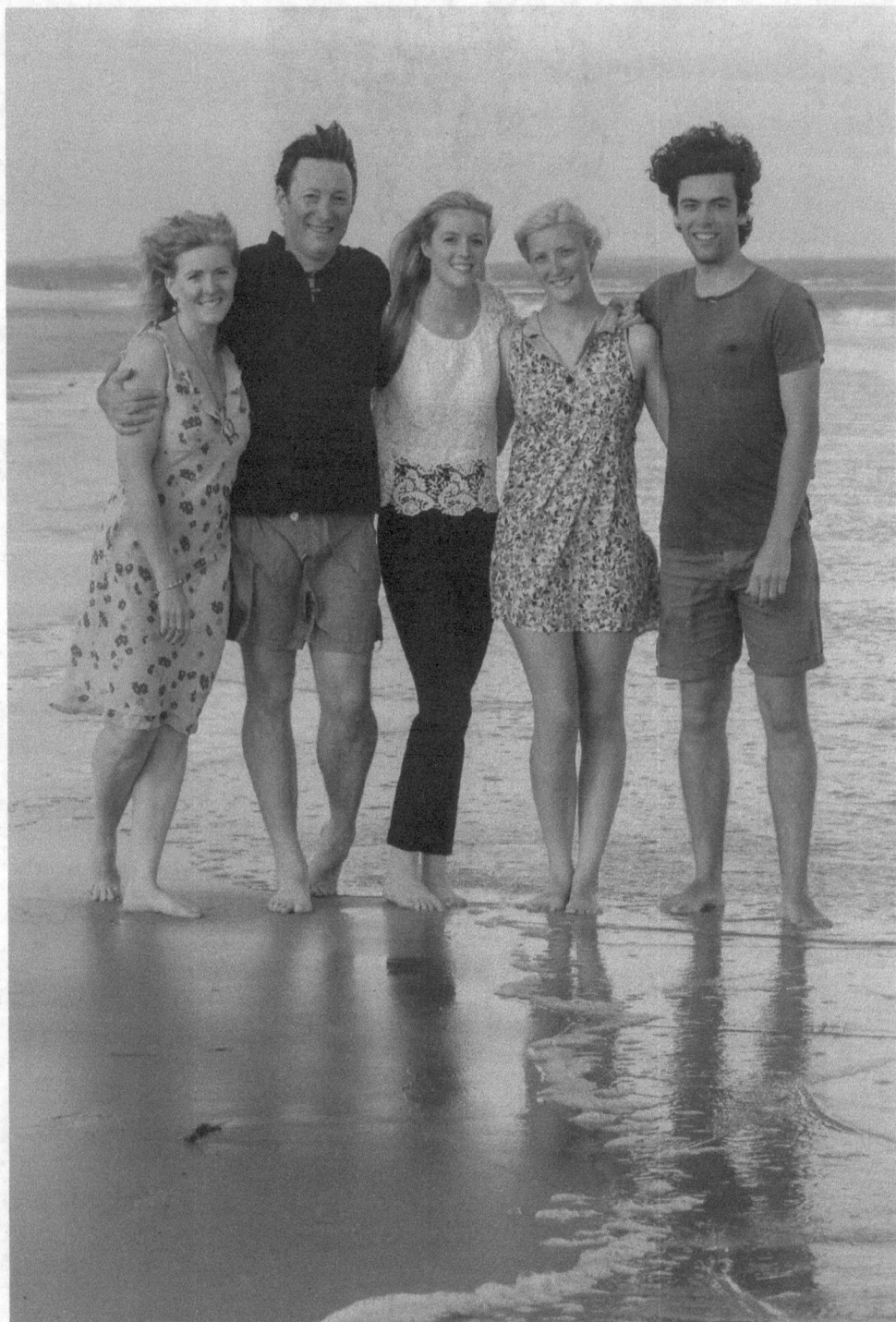

The surviving Frawleys on the beach at Jervis Bay, south coast of NSW, 2015.

26

ART OF SELF-DEFENCE

The individual has always had to struggle to keep from being overwhelmed by the tribe. If you try it, you will be lonely often, and sometimes frightened. But no price is too high to pay for the privilege of owning yourself.

— Friedrich Nietzsche

As Malachy's year in Ireland progressed, he moved from the small class of six to a larger class, combining the third and fourth grades into one. The social expansion this entailed was something of a relief for Malachy, whose outsider status was starkly obvious within the small group. Ruby, the school principal, taught the blended class. At first she was unsure how to react to Mac's willingness to speak his mind in class. Maggie had an uncomfortable interview, with Ruby describing him as bordering on insolence. Her response was a passionate defence of our son, explaining the degree of hardship he had faced, his courage, and the indomitable good nature and enthusiasm of the boy. To her credit Ruby stepped back from the initial discord, and developed a genuine enjoyment of Malachy's humour, and his oblique view of the ordinary. Malachy in turn liked and respected Ruby, responding well to her light-hearted yet firm teaching style. Amongst the students was a boy marked as different by an autistic spectrum disorder, apparently beyond the understanding of most of his peers, but not unfamiliar to Malachy, who had been friends with a boy 'on the spectrum' in Nowra.

Malachy's classmate was prone to unforeseen behavioural eruptions. Whether it was prior experience, their mutual outsider status or an innate quality in Malachy, but he was at ease with the child's eccentric unpredictability. At ease wasn't an apt description for the day Malachy arrived home with his forehead split open as a result of one of his friend's eruptions. In a sudden fit of disgruntlement, the boy hurled his note-binder blindly over his shoulder, the corners of the folder crashing into the face of the student seated behind. Quite rightly, Ruby was at pains to make a full explanation and apology to us for the injuries. A school's duty of care to a frail, disabled nine-year-old boy always runs to protecting them from acts of violence, even more so acts so completely lacking in cause or provocation. In our case there was the added complexity that if Malachy required surgical remedy, he wasn't like any other child you could pin down and stitch without fear of repercussion—there were heightened risks with regard to bleeding, infection, and risks to circulation while under anaesthetic. The risks were pertinent in so far as the forehead is cosmetically important, there's no hiding a scar in this region, and this one promised to be jagged and unsightly.

Malachy's response to the drama could be summarised as, 'I know he didn't mean anything by it, so it's okay. And besides, doesn't Harry Potter have a jagged scar down his forehead?' Case closed, nothing to see here, folks.

It would be an exaggeration to suggest this incident inspired Malachy's enrolment in Waterford Martial Arts (WMA), but somewhere around this time Maggie embarked on involving the children in what would prove to be one of our fondest memories of Waterford life. Yes, self-defence served as a potentially useful life skill for our puny son, but also offered hope of a sporting activity that could be modified to his limited aerobic capacity. Given how stir-crazy we could get with the slower pace of our rural existence, it also met the criteria for simply being something to do.

The Grandmaster of the school was a fearsomely large giant of a man, John McGrath, whose handshake enveloped my size eight fist as if it were that of a small child, as he towered over my mere six feet two inches. He impressed every bit as much with the discipline of his teaching and the lofty expectations he set for his pupils, as with his size. The theoretically desired inner calm of Eastern self-defensive arts was at the forefront in the school's teaching, reinforced by the temperament of its staff. This helped draw a wide range of young people to the floor, two or three times each week. Some came to progress skills in their chosen sport, others to build solidarity with like-minded friends who had stumbled on this secret font of confidence, and others seemed to have the classic Charles Atlas motivation—the traces of kicked sand subliminally being brushed from their faces as they rehearsed their future responses to bullying.

We needed to work through the way Malachy's limitations could be managed, both his poor exertion and his vulnerability to heavy impact. As you would expect his mixture of physical vulnerability with an engaging headstrong personality touched the heart of big John McGrath who found ways to adjust to these limitations and seemed to bring a special intent to his mentoring. It was lovely to watch this agile giant, whose arms each must have almost matched Malachy's weight, interacting with this tiny lad and bringing his charisma to bear on the task of inspiring belief that with time, and hard work, Malachy could be stronger, fitter and more confident. We hoped he would learn to escape from or terminate conflict.

The much-loved Teenage Mutant Ninja Turtles had previously triggered Mac's interest in the martial arts, so whatever gaps appeared in what his body could achieve, his imagination could fill as required.

One memorable feature of our involvement with Waterford Martial Arts was the teacher known to the children as Mr Fitzgerald. He was an Irishman of average size, whose many tattoos hinted at his rumoured history as an impecunious graduate of the school of hard knocks. His appearance would probably inspire apprehension if you spotted him in a dark alleyway. Regardless of how low he'd sunk (or not) before his apparent salvation through dedication to

Art of self-defence

martial arts, he certainly looked as if he had plenty of street cred. His manner with students was a delight to behold. Mr Fitzgerald was perfect in his movements, was emphatic in the didactic components, and encouraged the children to work hard and maintain dedication. He also had a passion for using what medical practitioners would refer to as 'normalisation' in describing the proper use of defensive art. He might for example say, 'So, in the next scenario, you are attending an ATM, a man approaches you with a knife. A VERY COMMON SITUATION...' Or, 'You are exiting your car and someone pulls a gun, A VERY COMMON SITUATION...'

We couldn't resist turning our thoughts to all the horrible things Mr Fitzgerald deemed very common, and what statistical level this equated with, but it was clear he was dedicated to protecting us in a world where abduction, throat slitting and gunshot wounds all nestled in the category 'Very Common Situations'.

Late in our Irish sojourn there was an opportunity for the children to undertake grading, where under external scrutiny by a visiting Grandmaster, they would each have to demonstrate proficient attainment of the skill level expected. This included enduring some demanding exercise routines, exemplary demonstration of a designated pattern of manoeuvres and skills and participation in suitably matched sparring. The grading took the greater part of a whole day, very arduous for the higher-grade applicants who were required to participate in each round of exercise leading up to their own formal grading.

The day was made entertaining by demonstrations of a fabulous range of skills by students and their masters alike. There were some terrific displays of numchuck and combat pole skills, and keenly awaited exhibitions by Mr Fitzgerald and John McGrath. We hoped upon hope for a 'Very Common Situation' to need defusing, allowing us to watch in stunned silence as Mr Fitzgerald took apart an assailant with his bare hands, as we were suitably convinced he would.

When the lights dimmed, we were surprised to see Mr Fitzgerald flowing around the floor space to the tinkling sounds of oriental

140

music, demonstrating a flawless, peaceful routine of Tai Chi. Those knife-wielding fiends would keep their limbs for one more day.

The climax of the show was a demonstration by the giant Sensei, John McGrath. In warm-up, a telephone book was torn in half in one go, thick blocks were broken and then he staged two dramatic tests.

First up, John was presented with a horseshoe, the rigid steel nature of which was demonstrated by banging against a nearby stand and the useless efforts of audience members to deform its shape by brute manipulation. With fanfare, the horseshoe was handed to John, who proceeded to twist its ends in opposing directions, deforming the unyielding structure to resemble a great thick segment of twisted coat hanger.

Next to the stage came a thick block of timber, mounted atop two vertical supports at waist height to the performer. Wedged between the supports, abutting the underside of the block of timber, was a party balloon. In John's hand was a thick six-inch nail, just long enough to penetrate the chunk of wood. The lights were dimmed, and once the music built to a crescendo; to the gasps of the crowd, John pounded that nail using only his hand through four inches of wood, bursting the balloon with the desired thunderclap of noise. The crowd roared with delight. We felt sure our children were learning in the right place at the feet of this man, part magician, part monster!

At the close of the day we met with Mr McGrath, complimenting him on the presentation and thanking him for his guidance of our children during their time in Ireland. Recognising he may not have another opportunity, he drew Malachy to his side and said, 'I want to give you something.' From a box, John drew the hardened steel sculpture that had once been a horseshoe. 'I'm giving this to you for now. Work hard and don't lose your belief. When you have returned this horseshoe to its original shape, then I want you to send it back to me.'

Mac was honoured to accept the memento. John's commission to exhibit strength and self-belief was not wasted on him.

27

WINTER SOLSTICE

People don't notice whether it's winter or summer when they're happy.

— Anton Chekhov

As the year wore on, we did as much travel as time and our other commitments allowed, both within Ireland, and to nearby countries. We saw castles and cliffs and caves, and the eerie wasteland of Ireland's Burren,[9] amongst many beautiful features; and came to love Ireland, warts, wetness and all.

We learnt to see the weather as our enemy and our teacher, learning to stare down its bitter challenge with stoic resistance. Emotion was both dulled by the constancy of drizzle and cold, heightened by the fondness that rare glimpses of sun produced. At any sign of sunshine, we learnt to look sideways in the knowledge there'd be a rainbow to dazzle with its precise optical beauty.

We found the Emerald Isle distinguished by its cosiness, as people seek to make the retreat indoors more appealing. The Irish excel in food preparation, with an emphasis on hearty, cockle-warming dishes. A sense of tradition attends the careful preparation of stews and pies, and seasonal treats. As the weather turned colder in the build-up to Christmas, we discovered varieties of mulled wine, and found the simple pleasure of warm drinks was heightened by

---

9   A vast cracked pavement of glacial-era rock formations, limestone cliffs and caves in County Clare, southwest Ireland.

contrast with the elements. Maggie enrolled in a course through one of the local caterers to learn the ancient art of the traditional Irish Christmas dinner. This would lead to the staging of one of the most resonant episodes of family togetherness in the raising of our children.

Expectation built through advent as the kitchen, always a hive of activity, bubbled into newfound productivity, with novel smells and sounds changing from one day to the next. Rum-soaked pudding took a turn, before passing to cake. A ham was cured from scratch and a turkey primed, dressed and basted for its one great day on the calendar. Adding to the excitement, our thoughts had turned to home, just a few short weeks away. We also had some visitors booked in. A family from Nowra were coming to stay after Christmas and the children yearned for the company of old friends.

The year had been long. There had been periods of loneliness and of financial strain. There had been disappointment and discovery, success and failure. Through much of it we'd had only each other as company; an intense nuclear family focus. That is a two-edged sword—good for children needing attention, not so much if you needed a break from your parents. Tensions had simmered from time to time as in any year, but there was nowhere for any of us to hide from each other. Heart-to-heart dialogue came and went, sometimes leaving a vague pall over the household. Now there was a lightening of the atmosphere. A clearing of the clouds. We had the approach of a home summer, reunions with friends and a return to the life-bringing sunshine of the temperate New South Wales south coast.

After a slow start the generosity and graciousness of many of the Waterford locals had us feeling more at home. In particular, we were welcomed by the people involved with the track and field club we took part in, and when my clinic opened in the September, we had more of a social context. The hardships of starting from scratch were fading away when the time came to return home. Having finally found our feet, the question of another year arose, briefly, before being dispelled. Home, on balance, was too enticing.

We came to the table that Christmas light of heart, replete with the many enjoyments of the year past, proud to have nearly survived our grand adventure and excited to reclaim our stalled lives south of the Shoalhaven River. Having no commitments beyond our tiny nuclear family, this Christmas was unlike any that had gone before. There would be no rush to the Extravagant Noble Family Feast for lunch, with its annual scramble to the Massive Extended Frawley Dinner.

Just dinner for six. No one to please but ourselves.

Malachy had proven himself hardier than expected in the face of Ireland's notoriously dreary weather and we'd managed to get through the whole year without dragging him to a doctor. He showed no signs of being deflated by the limitations of his small school network and had added some Irish quirkiness to his casual banter. He would return to Year 4 at St Michael's school far more worldly than he had left, one year earlier.

He was aided in this by Seamus, who shared his amusement at the exaggerated accents and mannerisms of the locals. Seamus's first year of high school had been interesting. He didn't have much social life to speak of, finding the school networks apparently too well-established to expand in his direction. An aptitude for language had seen him excel in German class. He had needed to become more independent, negotiating the public transport system to and from our remote farmhouse. Seamus had also found what it was like to coat himself in inches of icy mud, part of the weekly ritual of rugby training. He'd had the novel experience of having a match cancelled because the sheets of ice were too sharp and might lacerate the boys. Year 8 at a new high school beckoned from the antipodes.

Niamh had shared an upstairs bedroom with Malachy through the year, her equivalent of Year 5. She had gathered friends at every turn and proven a tremendous asset to the regional athletics club. Schoolwork contained some surprises, including ample homework. In that sphere, Niamh discovered an aptitude for numbers, as well as enjoying her mandatory Irish language (Gaelic) classes. We all enjoyed encouraging her to perform a lilting Gaelic poem she had rote-learnt for a performance at her village school.

The year had contained some flat patches for Imogen, who gave us our first experience of the perils of teen transformation. Her gentle nature made her slow to bond with the locals. The local girls' tendency to do more singing, drinking, and fighting, and to cake on more makeup made them appear so different in their culture and manner from her childhood friends, but by the winter break Imogen had formed enough of a network to make the year worthwhile. Her year would be capped off by a visit from one of her best friends from Australia, Hannah, whose family squeezed into Bob's Lodge for a short stay and joined us on some regional travels. The close proximity of our lifestyle in Ireland becomes more valuable now in hindsight. It was the last year Imogen would live at home, having enrolled in boarding school at Loreto Normanhurst for 2009.

Maggie was always looking for constructive ways to pass the time, given the bureaucratic barriers of paid work. As the year drew to a close, she had enrolled in the cooking classes directed at the Christmas season. By that time, I had regular long shifts at the SwiftCare clinic, and my year was beginning to drag on a bit.

All six of us were ready to live it up for Christmas as we converged on the cottage kitchen at Bob's Lodge.

Maggie's weeks of preparation ensured the feast spread before us was superb as sprouts jostled with chestnuts, which blended with bread sauce. Apple sauce for this, cranberry for that. Each item through a combination of skill and grace was perfect in taste and presentation, the whole affair elevated to mythic status by our shared sense of accomplishment and festive bonhomie. At a point in the meal, I felt a deep calm diffuse through the room. I'm sure Maggie felt it too. The volume dimmed. We looked around the room, its warm air permeated with love. Time stopped, and the six people we most treasured soaked in the suspended moment. That moment coalesced all the best of our lives to date. That moment yelled to the heavens: Life Is Beautiful!

Perhaps we knew we'd never have this time again: childhood must end, and siblings move apart. Parents grow less useful as independence blooms.

I'd have bottled that day and that moment if I could. As it is, I'm content to put what remains of it on this page. I can visit it here in print and in memory.

As we basked in the glow of our own happiness, donned paper hats and shared stupid jokes from bon-bons, Malachy piped up with a declaration: 'Everyone, I have an announcement. From now on … we'll have this meal every Christmas.'

Everyone paused briefly to concur, and further agreed, and loudly declared it was the Best Christmas Ever, before resuming our feast, secure in the knowledge that love was at the core of our family life and the future promised more such occasions.

Maggie and I caught eyes, contentment beaming across the table to meet in the middle. It was tough, but we got there. A treasure trove of shared memories had seeped and burrowed its way deep into our collective family life.

28

(ANTI) HEROES IN PRINT

*Become aware of what is in you. Announce it, pronounce it,
produce it and give birth to it.*

— Meister Eckhart

The return from Ireland in 2009 brought some changes to the
pattern of our lives. I resumed at my old practice, relieved to
enjoy the freedom of being the boss once more after the relative
subservience I had endured as a travelling bit-worker. I swiftly
became as busy as I'd ever been with both patient care and my
responsibilities as an owner.

Maggie's role as state manager of HeartKids had passed to a
woman who was a survivor of childhood heart disease, and the
national body remained under the stewardship of Neil McWhannell,
the CEO who had been appointed in 2007. It was a source of great
satisfaction to both of us to realise we had made the contribution
we had, and though we had moved on, the HeartKids movement
was going from strength to strength. Maggie resumed her teaching
career, adding another degree to her list of accomplishments, by
switching from primary to secondary teaching.

Our youngest child got on with the business of growing up. He
would gradually have to move from childhood to teenager. Time
and hormones would do some of the work. Limited as he was in
physical ability, Mac focused on the development of his mind.

Malachy brought a particular intensity to his engagement
with fictional characters. He discussed them with great relish,

assuming his audience would share his fascination with the topic at hand. The attributes of the characters were described, as if extolling the virtues of an old friend. Frequently I felt inclined to check Malachy's understanding, along the lines of, 'You know he's not a real person, right?' For his part, Malachy seemed to ascribe only limited relevance to the question of their existence. He brought highly sensitive analysis to the nuance that authors instilled in their creations, revelling in the ability of the writer to build complex characters. No effort went to waste on this receptive reader. Imaginary people were every bit as influential for Malachy as real ones.

Reading time then, was spent in the company of 'friends'. This presented no problem when the company Malachy kept was of a suitable calibre. The always earnest and charming Harry Potter, for example, was the sort of company any parent would be delighted for their child to keep; free of guile, modest despite grand accomplishments, loyal to a fault, fair in judgment and willing to forgive. What's more, Harry Potter always put protecting others ahead of his personal needs, his life at the service of humanity, using his genius always for the greater good. Villains and heroes of old were perfectly designed to encourage a gifted child to use their genius for good, instead of evil. No sane child would model themselves on arch nemeses like Lex Luthor. In traditional vein, J.K. Rowling's beloved teen hero brought an innocent, brave, innately wise presence into the post Generation Y world. On the cusp of high school life, Malachy, swept along with most of his generation, could do a lot worse than embracing the values of Harry Potter's altruistic heroism. To my great joy I had a son who liked to share the process of search and discovery.

It fascinated me that Malachy could distil and explain essential traits from the characters created by authors such as Daniel Handler, Derek Landy, Rick Riordan, Eoin Colfer and Christopher Paolini, who feature among the series sitting proudly huddled on the shelf in Malachy's room. As a collective, these writers and many others emerging around the turn of the twenty-first century, either whittle away at, or completely abandon the once obvious dividing line between 'goodies' and 'baddies'. In their pages, 'baddies' are found to be not all bad, and the heroes, well, didn't we always suspect they were too good to be true? Mixed motivations and complex ambitions swirled around the reader in a post-modern maze of moral decision-making, with the outcome of a wrestle between fear and courage not always predictable. Reluctant heroes were all very well, but how should we feel about greedy, shallow, or positively nasty ones? If our hero is sired by a god, surely they will be faultless? What might we learn from the life and times of a living-dead skeleton with a penchant for black humour?

Eragon, from Paolini's *Inheritance Cycle*, had formative impact for Malachy, more for its author's background than for any post-modern qualities. The captivating epic heroic tale is more of a traditional clash of good and evil, but stunning in Malachy's eyes was the fact that as he penned the first instalment of the saga, Christopher Paolini was only 15 years old. Such precociousness in Malachy's view brought achievement of a successful magnum opus into the realms of not just the remotely possible in an imagined distant future, but attainable in a span of mere years rather than decades.

There was a compelling logic to Malachy's interpretation. Why wait to grow up in order to be what you want to be when you grow up?

Marking the other end of the spectrum, distinctively anti-epic and relentlessly postmodern, Malachy was hugely entertained by the *Lemony Snicket* series. The author Daniel Handler titled the books, *A Series of Unfortunate Events,* and goes to delicious lengths to warn potential readers of the horrible content of his tales of woe. So awful and dire are his warnings, it is impossible not to plunge in and start reading. Bleak tales of hardship, loss and dastardly child abuse spring lightly off the page, decorated with all manner of experimental literary devices, darkly twisted humour and a self-consciously intrusive narrator. Malachy would laugh out loud, and often feel compelled to reread exceptional passages for my edification. The powerful presence of the author within the tale impressed Mac, elevating Handler into his pantheon of model writers.

Self-referential black humour is very much the stock-in-trade of Derek Landy's *Skulduggery Pleasant*; it would become a regular feature of Malachy's writing. The ironic flavour of mocking superhero banter during combat, heroic self-deprecation and off-hand responses to cataclysmic events, all seemed to match Malachy's humour to perfection. I took great pleasure from following up his enthusiasm by reading the books he loved and finding in their pages the double joy of my own reading combined with a sense of how I saw the works moved inside Malachy. With his guidance, I could track the inspiration he derived from his own literary travels. I had a sense that he was sharing with me not just stories he liked, but a map of his mental 'wiring'. As I read, I loved not just the book at hand, but the impact I imagined it had in the expanding world of my cherished son.

One happy development along this post-modern explosion of possibilities was Malachy's acquisition of a fascination for the ancient world. The mythology of ancient Greece and Rome was brought to life for Malachy in the works of Rick Riordan, the creator of *Percy Jackson*. The canon of Western thought and literary achievement has long held that classical understanding offers potentially infinite insight and wisdom to the learned. Rightly or wrongly, a certain intellectual pride attaches to classical scholarship, the recognition of references to the mythological lessons of our forebears being deemed to bring a beautiful symmetry to the refined mind. How brimming with irony it is to realise the door to the world of classical refinement was opened through the low-brow mechanism of a best-selling children's novel? Percy Jackson, it turns out, unbeknownst to himself was a halfling Greek god, plunged into the world of his forebears by circumstances beyond his contemporary angst-ridden teenage existence, dragging both him and Malachy into the pantheistic ancient world. Malachy's world view and his literary imagination would now be further stimulated and nurtured by an increasing knowledge of history, and exposure to the universal moral dilemma of cultural mythology.

Malachy's reading spanned not only his thirst for knowledge his desire to write and the sheer pleasure of reading but also contributed to his emerging sense of self—Who am I going to be?

On that question, possibly the greatest influence Malachy shared with me was from an unexpected source, the work of the Irish author Eoin Colfer, creator of *Artemis Fowl*.

At one level Colfer's story is about growing up with all the potential of the individual captured on the cusp of adulthood, where it will lead is the great unknown. At another level there is a tale about greed, aspiration, moral decision-making, and the timeless struggle between good and evil. Artemis had qualities that appealed greatly to Malachy, either through identification or aspiration. They shared being 12 years old, being separated from their peers by virtue of innate characteristics and being ambitious for a life beyond the ordinary. Then there was stuff they didn't share, such as Artemis being a multimillionaire, a criminal mastermind, and ruthless to the point of sociopathy. Other than that, there was a bunch of qualities either up for grabs or open to interpretation, such as his advanced scheming ability, cynical insight into the workings of human nature, heedless disrespect for authority and imperious leadership style. Artemis complemented his personal attributes and exaggerated his distance from his peers with a keen sartorial sense, dressing far more formally than the average teen. These were qualities neither all good nor all bad, not clearly designed for rejection by the reader, but not truly suitable for wholesale adoption either. You could think of this as Artemis's potential sphere of influence over Malachy.

As we discussed and enjoyed the tale, I could sense Malachy's measuring of the character traits on show. I couldn't help but notice a hint of glee at the evil uses to which Artemis put his genius, a tone of admiration for his effrontery around teachers and police, and downright cockiness at the precociousness of carrying it all off at age twelve. More than a striking character, he was also a prodigy. Further, not content just to be prodigious, Artemis was a boy who dressed the part. We chuckled at the descriptions of this child antihero in a tailored three-piece suit and silk tie.

I am certain it is not entirely coincidental that acquaintance with these books was at its height when Malachy started his later famous predilection for ties. As a professional who mostly avoids ties, wearing one perhaps once or twice a year, it was a bit odd for me to arrive home from work and find myself underdressed to hang out with my teenage son.

Malachy may have been ignoring some of Artemis's own sage advice that, 'Confidence is ignorance. If you're feeling cocky, it's because there's something you don't know.' But I detected a growing sense of presence around Malachy, an increasing feeling of certainty about how he would like to project himself. How far he might go in testing his assuredness in the face of authority, or in allowing his genius to be put to dubious ends might be hard to measure, but a persona that said, 'I've arrived' had emerged.

There is a photograph taken at a family function at my parents' home that captures this evolutionary point in time. It's a relatively disorganised portrait of a group of children, of various ages, siblings and cousins called to look in the direction of a camera, each putting on their camera face with different levels of regard and interest. The image has served a long stint in the kitchen, attached to our fridge. Front and centre is Malachy, most formal of the group, a collared shirt with broad stripes, buttoned at the wrists, the neat collar the starting point for a tie of silk. He is the only person wearing a tie. The light seems to be trapped a little by his shirt, bringing his image to prominence, with his face intent on the camera.

Whether it is the formality of his apparel, his central position, the steel in his eyes, or a hint of authority in his posture, something about his look conveys importance, a feeling that he is central to the capture of this moment in time.

Malachy had a sense of moment. I don't know if he felt an urgency that others didn't. Maybe each moment of time was more precious from his vantage point.

29

PERSONAE GONE ROGUE

I liked pretending to be other people: I could reinvent myself, reinvent my own reality.

— Helena Bonham Carter

The English artist, Grayson Perry, contends that, 'The most beautiful and complex artwork that we can make is our identity'. Accepting this paradigm, Malachy's greatest artwork was surging ahead through his primary years. Powerful as they may be, books were far from the only formative influence on the sweeping canvas of personal identity. Becoming his future self was not a passive exercise in aging for this young man. Malachy sought out ideas and constantly imagined into shape a future worth aspiring to. Drawing from life as well as from fiction, Mac's gift of careful observation was helpful in putting together the elements of his emerging persona.

Ordinary childhood experiences would remain burdened by the limitations of his malformed heart. After returning to Australia there was a surge of enthusiasm for handball, a sport confined to a small court with little requirement for aerobic fitness. Timing and coordination were not beyond Malachy's feeble frame, so we dared to be swept along by his reports of some joy in the playground. The sporting opportunity Malachy so craved found a focus that wasn't obviously doomed to end in failure and tears, and the stories of hand-ball skirmishes, the struggle for ascendancy and the coping with defeat, briefly took on the drama others might associate with grand final football.

The tiny court does not isolate the game of handball from the earthly surrounds of the playground, and the argy-bargy of school pecking orders. It happened one day that Malachy encountered a standard yard nuisance, a bully who flung Malachy's ball across the yard, forcing him to have to fetch it, thus buying time for another group to invade the court. The bully was at least a little bit street-smart, but that didn't make him any smaller, or kinder. Mac struggled off to fetch, predictably taking much longer than the average child to return, labouring as he had to against a slight incline and a compromised heart. A challenge quietly suffered, at the cost of some distress, while he waited his turn to rejoin the game. Having rejoined, it happened again. Malachy let fly. Unable to physically match the bully he exclaimed, 'You are an imbecile!' and further told him how stupid he was and how he had nothing going for him except that he was bigger and that didn't stop him being a loser (or words to that effect).

The sequel to this event included Maggie and I observing Malachy's distress at seeing handball, this one pleasurable activity, tainted by the actions of a bully. In a surprising turn of events, we were stunned to be notified by the school that our son was a bully. We were told Malachy needed to learn not to use his superior mental agility to hurt other boys! We were shocked to realise the complete failure of some to recognise the truth of the exchange. It seemed remarkable that people didn't perceive the extent of Malachy's challenges, nor understand the genuine fragility of his dusky blue-pink body. Maybe Malachy coped too well to attract the deserved level of sympathy. Awareness remains a problem for sufferers—children's heart disease is a hidden scourge.

Outwardly, Mac coped very well and was thriving. Nonetheless the incident served to alert us to some flaws emerging in the canvas of personal identity. The well documented strain of day-to-day existence was spilling over into bursts of frustration. It may have been the first signs of the demon testosterone sparking Mac's anger, which seemed so uncharacteristic. It happened enough to be identified within the family as something akin to volcanic eruptions, earning our hero the nickname, Makatoa. An unfair reference in that the eruption of Mt Krakatoa is said to be the loudest noise in modern history.

The emotional weight of transforming into his future self, ensured Malachy suffered definitively human imperfection and uncertainty, and the requisite encounter with his own failings that marks the challenge of emerging into adulthood.

With frayed edges and dark moments, exclusion and physical constraints, perhaps the nascent masterpiece was something of a patchwork quilt. A splendid quilt needs splashes of colour to balance the darkness.

Enter 'Cousin Jarred' from New Zealand. This character sprang up as if from thin air one Saturday, to land on the sideline at one of Niamh's soccer games. Always content to create his own world within his bedroom, or the safety of home, Malachy suddenly took his imagination out in the field in the form of alter-ego Jarred. Malachy was clear in his request that we not blow his cover, but that on arrival at the game we introduce this creature in bright red wig, dark glasses, and hipster/pimp street wear as our nephew Jarred. Niamh for her part was every bit as adamant that she wanted nothing to do with the embarrassing weirdo and would not greet or refer to him. Malachy attended the game, spoke true 'fush and chup' speak for the duration, without anyone questioning his assumed identity. His first foray into alter ego was an almost unqualified success. Niamh's forgiveness would be slow in coming.

Streetwear such as Jarred's had its place, but when it came to fashions, Malachy had a taste for the timeless. A range of influences may have been at play, including the leanings of a Television character, Barney from the American sitcom *How I Met Your Mother*, who characteristically would wear nothing but fine suits. Malachy also had a father who was always somewhat anti-fashion and cultivated a dressed-down style from his teen years. Barney and friends won the culture war, as from the age of ten or eleven Mac was relentlessly drawn to 'suiting up' and wore at least a collar and tie to most social outings, heedless of peer influence or parental taste.

In the case of Malachy's clothes, despite their position well outside the norm for his age and era, I would share Hamlet's reservations about the idea that, 'Clothes maketh the Man', and certainly Malachy understood there must be substance added to his persona. With all the options open to an active agent in construction of an identity, how should one speak, and carry oneself, and balance humour with serious intent. Perhaps his imaginary world was where he combed over questions of the kind. We could see him absorbing, accruing and trialling new attributes almost week to week.

The manner of delivery Mac was evolving owed something to his love of stand-up comedy. Once discovered, this was a well he would return to draw from repeatedly, whether it was Lee 'Sweaty Comedian' Evans, or Dara O Briain, or Ross Noble, or his out-and-out favourite, the Englishman, Michael McIntyre—Malachy couldn't get enough. His computer screen 'me time' went into a phase of daily YouTube comedy, taking over from the once addictive war and empire games.

There didn't seem to be any down time in Mac's identity building creativity, as he adopted measured phrasing to deliver punchlines, or waxed lyrical about the latest offering from McIntyre, or a stylish retort by Skulduggery Pleasant or Artemis Fowl's latest fiendish venture. The classical battles between Greek gods as they wrestled for the soul of the human race occupied him. Their lofty themes inspired something in Mac, allowing his mind to soar where his body was unable. He ruminated about the things that motivated the gods or made these characters work, or that elevated one performer above their peers. Sometimes it seemed he was choosing the building blocks from which to fashion has own pathway to greatness.

The problem was time. The great unknown: how much time do I have?

Christopher Paolini, having penned *Eragon* at the tender age of 15 had set the benchmark for frenetically productive teen life. This intrigued and encouraged Malachy, who increasingly defined himself as a man in a hurry.

One way Malachy put it, addressing me by nickname, was this: 'D-Money, what I want to be is an author; I want to write stories. I just need to get published by the time I'm 16 so I can still be a child prodigy.'

The signature on his greatest of artworks, his hard-won identity, would need to be Malachy Frawley: Child Prodigy.

MALACHY'S MAGNUM OPUS

Esteban Devereaux's Adventure
Chapter Two
— Malachy Frawley 2013

Esteban woke up the next morning to the tuneful singing of whatever birds happened to be outside his window at that time. He was also feeling quite proud of himself. **I'll do that walk again tonight,** he thought, as he got out of his bed. He briefly looked in the mirror on his wall and laughed, amused at what going to bed with wet hair had done to him. Esteban had decided that washing in the morning was probably a better idea than washing at night a long time ago, but that didn't mean he enjoyed it as much. He practically stumbled out of his room and down the corridor that was lit up like Christmas from the early morning sun. He entered the kitchen and just stood there. His mum looked up from her Newspaper and his dad looked up from Esteban's Nintendo DS.

'Hey, Esteban,' they said, almost in unison.

'Morning.' Esteban went and sat down at the round table his parents were sitting at. 'What are you playing, dad?'

'Mario.'

'But that's mine.'

'Sssh, I'm concentrating ... Aw, you made me lose!'

'Sorry, dad, but it's still mine.'

'That's okay.'

Esteban made himself a bowl of cereal that he didn't recognise and when he was finished went back to his room. He threw on his ugly green uniform that consisted of a white, collared shirt, a green tie, a green blazer and white polyester pants which were so grass-stained they actually kind of matched his blazer, which was surprising because **nothing** should match a green **that** musty and hideous. As he put his bag on and lifted up his laptop that was in its case, which was much heavier than it should have been, he looked out the window. A great white light passed through the sky heading towards Esteban's house. Esteban was having trouble figuring out what it was when he realised that it was going to crash to the earth near to his house.

He walked outside into his weed-filled garden that desperately needed maintenance, and watched the strange white light fall through the sky just over the hill up from his house. The hill he had spent an hour walking up the previous day. He was going to head back inside when there was an earsplittingly loud noise that shook the ground, almost causing Esteban to fall over. At the same time there was a *HUGE* flash of searing white light that burst over the edge of the hill, rising over the horizon like a second sun, and then it faded into the bitterly cold morning winter air. *Alright,* thought Esteban, *Forget school, I'm climbing this hill, right here, right now!* Esteban dumped his bag and his weirdly heavy laptop and started to walk up the hill at a blistering pace ... which turned out to be a **terrible** idea as it was mere seconds before he had to sit down and have a rest. *Right,* he thought, *I'll just wait here and when I regain my breath, I'll just take it nice and slow, like a clever tortoise once did.*

He started his slow ascent up the slope, and out of the corner of his mismatched eyes he saw a figure across the road heading up the hill a little behind him. He turned his head and fist-pumped inside his mind. Across the road from him was Lyris, the extremely talented and good looking, not to mention athletic all-star, girl from his school. She was wearing the same hideous uniform as he was, but her pants were somehow completely white and she seemed to pull it off, a feat thought impossible by Esteban. She had blonde-brown wavy hair that cascaded over her shoulders and down her back. Her eyes were an astonishingly blue colour, and she sported a pair of slick, red-tinged glasses that really accentuated her eyes. Esteban was quite good friends with her and crossed the road to talk to her. As he walked across the wet, dark tar he marvelled at her immaculately white pants and wondered how she did it. **She probably gets them washed properly**, he thought to himself. Esteban's parents hand washed everything for a reason he did not know. **Maybe**, he thought, **They think they're too indie for a washing machine or maybe they're just weird.** 'Probably the latter,' he accidentally said aloud.

'What?' said Lyris.

Esteban jumped. 'Nothing,' he said.

'I could have sworn you said something.'

'Nope, not me. Must have been the ... ah ... the birds?' he asked hopefully.

'Birds don't talk, Esteban.' said Lyris.

'Some do!'

Lyris paused. 'You're so weird.'

'Why, thank you.' Esteban continued up the hill mentally kicking himself in the face. 'Sooo,' he said, 'why are you walking up the hill at this hour of the morning?'

'Oh, you know, to find out what the HUGE explosion and flash of light was about—you might have noticed it.'

'That's what I'm doing as well.' Esteban said, clearly failing to read her sarcasm. Esteban struggled up the hill, desperately trying to keep up with Lyris and her graceful strides that were fast leaving him behind.

'Can we please stop and rest?' he asked.

She stared at him.

'What?'

'I'm sorry, I need a rest.'

'Okay.'

To be continued...

PART 3

YOUNG MAN

Surviving and thriving

30

MOBILITY

I don't work on a project unless I believe that it will dramatically improve life for a bunch of people.

— Dean Kamen

The family had to constantly innovate to preserve Malachy's mobility over the years.

The stroller served us well, until at five years of age, Mac had to declare himself too old to be happy being seen pushed in a baby's carriage. Our original baby back-pack played a key role in our Australian road trip, in 2004. It was later replaced by a sturdier model, but became unwieldy by 2008, when Malachy's legs grew so long, they dragged on the ground.

That situation called for something lightweight, portable, and propelled without much effort from Malachy. The ideal solution also wouldn't require me or another helper to exert themselves beyond their current fitness level. A heart attack for the helper would really defeat the purpose.

During a camping trip a 40-litre water container gave me an idea. Wrestling as I needed to, to fill the container at a distant tap then lug it, with repeated rest stops back to our campsite inspired me to make use of Seamus's old skateboard. By resting the barrel on the board, I found I could glide the 40-kilo mass back to our site with only modest exertion. I figured the method could be applied to a 40-kilo human.

Malachy tried his balance on the board. It was fine; he just needed someone there to push.

We tested a similar technique on a family weekend in Sydney, using a collapsible scooter. We were staying in Walsh Bay, near the famous Rocks' district. From Walsh Bay the jewels of Sydney city are all within walking distance for the able-bodied. It's quite a long walk if you stay on the flat, following the road all the way around the point; but much shorter if you slice straight from Hickson Road to the tail end of George Street. We ambled at our usual family speed dictated by Malachy, with me nudging him forward by the small of his back on the scooter. Maggie spotted a place to cut east under the Sydney Harbour Bridge towards Circular Quay, where the street life is bustling and atmospheric. We stood and stared up, and up, at a daunting tower of stairs, as Malachy let out a prolonged groan, 'No, not stairs. Guys, no, I hate stairs.'

Unfazed, the others stepped forward and took turns to piggyback their brother. First Imogen, then Seamus took Mac on board, managing more than 40 steps each before depositing him on the top landing. Then another groan went up. The steps had led us to the base of a steep hill. Niamh, herself barely bigger than Malachy, urged him to climb on. She charged upwards with Malachy as passenger, showing strength well beyond the slightness of her frame. With guts and determination, she forged doggedly 50 metres to flatter road ahead. There, Maggie and I continued pushing him forward through the light pedestrian traffic with suitable ease.

The combination of skateboards and devoted siblings was a winner.

Another innovation of note was the 'caravan' bike which afforded Mac his only chance to take part in family bike rides. It was a single-wheeled attachment onto the seat post of my bicycle, allowing me to tow him along. Mac had the option of contributing some (rare!) pedalling at his leisure. With the caravan attachment Mac got to share the invigorating rush of air on his face as we gathered speed down hills.

Like every other device we tried, Malachy's use of the caravan bike kept him dependent on somebody else's help to get around.

Every other device that is, except the Segway, invented by Dean Kamen.

Dean Kamen is far from a household name, but the man is something of a hero to me. The son of a *MAD* magazine artist, Kamen has a long string of inventions to his name. He invented the means by which lights blare at you in time to the music at rock concerts. He also invented medical infusion pumps, and an amazing prosthetic arm, with nearly all the capabilities of a real human arm. He also invented the self-balancing iBOT wheelchair which can carry a passenger up a set of stairs unassisted. The iBOT is so agile it was nicknamed 'Fred Upstairs' likening its deftness to the dancing of Fred Astaire. The gyroscopic mechanism hidden in the chair is the purest gem of engineering invention. A similar mechanism is used in Kamen's later invention: the 'Segway PT'.

The Segway is a two-wheeled personal transporter device, with foot plates and a steering column topped with a set of handlebars. The machine balances itself, leaving the rider to dictate the speed by moving their weight back or forward on the footplates, and to steer by tilting the handlebars. The rider travels almost completely without personal strain.

Inspired by its possibilities, in November 2010 HeartKids purchased a Segway for Malachy to use. It was to have a huge personal impact on Malachy.

My memory of the day Malachy first rode his Segway is vivid. We had both been excited by the possibilities it offered, but Malachy was apprehensive about the coordination involved in riding the thing. As we waited at the old train yard at Homebush Bay for our appointed lesson time, he was a bundle of nerves. Maggie and I sought to sooth his anxiety though we, too, were a little uncertain whether Mac's little-used coordination would be up to the task.

Graham, the Segway instructor, was at pains to explain in great detail all the safety considerations. He emphasised at length that the Segway was, 'not a toy', and was potentially dangerous in the wrong hands. Mac's knees shook and we feared he'd be scared off before risking the dire consequences he'd been warned of.

After some cajoling, he placed his feet, anxiously, on the footplates. The machine lurched back and forward as if to expel him. Forward, back, forward, back it bucked, with each lurch thankfully smaller than the one preceding it, until it steadied. Graham held the handles and fixed Malachy with a stare. 'Okay, you see it's steady now. You were trying too hard to balance. Remember, it will balance for you.'

We would later see almost every first-time Segway user start with a bunch of back and forward lurches, working too hard to control the self-correcting machine.

Once steadied, Malachy was guided through some slow careful practice at turning first left, then right, a little bit of backwards, and a little bit of forwards. Suddenly, grasping the technique, he shot off across the fields with his instructor and disappeared from view. Neil, the CEO of HeartKids, commandeered another Segway, lunged back and forward, and careered off to join in the fun. A sponsor who had helped with the purchase was on hand with her camera and managed to capture some beautiful photographs as Mac and Neil together delighted in the novelty and sheer joy of effortless propulsion.

So thrilled was Malachy that the next day he suited up in a full black lounge suit, complete with tie, just to take the Segway for a spin on our street.

It is hard to describe the new freedom Malachy enjoyed through the simple addition of independent mobility. It gave him the normal opportunities of childhood exploration as pushbikes did for the more able-bodied. Having always been denied such 'normality', Malachy relished his new freedom of movement so hungrily you could feel a rush of excitement every time he shot off through the front gate.

Nowra became a place of discovery as he unearthed and named all sorts of interesting alleys and buildings, and joined in an imaginary game in which dark conspiracies were housed and scattered around the town. With his great mate PJ, they developed an elaborate scheme of invented problems and challenges, all of which required them to 'Seg' around town in pursuit of a solution. His imaginary world had finally burst through the four walls of his bedroom. The physical world shrank to become accessible. Malachy, the exploring hero in his private narrative, gradually sped further afield.

Making very good use of the 30-kilometre range of the machine, Malachy was now able to visit his friends as well as allowing me to go riding with him rather than needing to tow him. The speed limiter of the device meant my mountain bike could fly down the hills much faster than the Segway, but the Segway didn't tire on the uphills the way I did, so the race was well-matched.

To my surprise, the laws of New South Wales don't allow Segways on either roads or footpaths though we never encountered a local police officer who wanted to be the one to ban a child with heart disease from visiting his friends.

We did encounter red tape on a family excursion to Jamberoo Action Park—famously advertised as the place 'where you control the action'. Most children in our region loved the park, but it was never accessible to Malachy by virtue of its steep hillside setting. We built up the excitement of the attraction for Mac, buzzing about the Segway's capacity to deliver him to the top of the waterslides and bobsled runs, where gravity would deliver the fun.

Arriving at the gate, two security guards barred Mac's entry. They barked at him that no vehicles were allowed in. Mac was almost in tears at the shock rejection.

In a flash, my flight or fight hormones kicked in and I lost my cool. My usual calm disposition evaporated in desperate anger as I saw Malachy's hopes cut down so unexpectedly. Watching his lifetime of exclusions had clearly made me highly sensitive on my son's behalf. Surprising myself, I sprang aggressively in the direction of the burly gentlemen. Anger fought briefly with rational consideration as I recalled every bad outcome I'd ever had at the hands of petty authority. I found my inner diplomat.

Keen not to embarrass Malachy with a scene, I asked for a quiet word with the guards, explaining, 'I'm sorry, you don't understand, but this is not a toy, this is the equivalent of a wheelchair. I am sure you allow people to enter with wheelchairs? My son has a serious heart disease.'

I knew I was rushing the words and was not at my most charming. In my despair, I had enough sense not to make the men feel I was challenging their authority. To their credit the case for Malachy was won and the rules were bent, allowing him to enjoy a wonderful outing.

The gift of mobility would go on to contribute to many wonderful days.

31

PRIDE

We want progress in medicine to be clear and unequivocal, but of course it rarely is. Every new treatment has gaping unknowns – for both patients and society – and it çan be hard to decide what to do about them.

— Atul Gawande

Imogen went off to boarding school in Sydney, in January 2009 after we arrived home from Ireland, while Seamus started at St John's, the high school Maggie worked at. Niamh and Malachy rejoined their old friends at St Michael's, the parish primary school. It was a period of consolidation, with Mac continuing his good run after not needing a doctor through our whole time away.

Malachy acquired the Segway in the spring of the next year, 2010. A short while later, the staff at HeartKids made contact to ask whether Malachy, then ten, would help with some marketing. 'Yes', he was willing to make a film to raise money for the charity. The request was in relation to a Commonwealth Bank charity promotion called Community Seeds. A range of charities competed for donations using short films about their cause. Internet users voted for the most impressive campaign. For every vote, the bank would donate a dollar to the designated charity. As a bonus, the charity attracting the highest number of votes would receive an additional donation of $25,000.

For the HeartKids movie Malachy was filmed undergoing a stress test; walking on a treadmill until exhaustion claimed him. Confrontingly, exhaustion derailed him less than two minutes into the effort.

He was then filmed using his Segway around a track in a park. Malachy is seen gliding effortlessly in defiance of gravity around a path in a suburban park. Close-up shots from a mounted camera show obvious glee as wisps of hair blows back in the breeze and the branches of gum trees whiz by overhead. The resulting short film included candid expressions of Malachy's pure delight and gratitude. The Segway symbolised the transformative potential of HeartKids. Through the vignette Malachy swept all before him, topping the vote count on the website, securing maximum prize money and the jackpot bonus for HeartKids.

Malachy felt rightly satisfied with his latest contribution to the cause. Maggie and I beamed with pleasure to see him so engaged and so happy.

One Saturday afternoon in August 2011 Malachy, Maggie, and I made our way to Sydney's Hilton Hotel. The ballroom was abuzz with expectation when we arrived. The nervous electricity of last-minute preparations permeated the air as dedicated volunteers buzzed around, setting up for HeartKids' Tiny Tickers Ball. There were 55 exquisitely decorated banquet tables receiving their finishing touches. Malachy and I had a specific part in preparation, for our young son was a formal guest speaker. After months of preparation, any untimely hiccup could now wreak their havoc, and it showed on some of the faces!

Our friend, Mary, the organiser of the Tiny Tickers Ball, was sweating on the final arrangements and needed to ask something of me. One of the performers had cracked his head on the floor in final rehearsal and needed a doctor at short notice. I rushed off, delaying Malachy's run-through while I searched the building for the injured dancer. I gave the dancer the thumbs-up to proceed, while the clock ticked down to showtime.

Back at the ballroom I tracked down the event's Master of Ceremonies, who was to elucidate Malachy's story through an interview on stage. Simon Reeve was a delightful media personality, well known to the audience as a loyal supporter of children with heart disease. Simon, like us, had a Heart Kid—his son Sam. Simon and Malachy had bonded years earlier when Simon had done some documentary filming of Malachy around one of his operations. Malachy had an enthusiasm to resume their friendship for the proceedings.

In the bustle, Simon clearly had a full night's agenda to prepare, Malachy's interview being nestled in with auctioneering, silent auctions, speeches from a cardiologist, a parent and representatives of HeartKids. There were also to be two or three rounds of entertainment from the dance troupe. The need to bustle was clear as we sat down to plan our time in the spotlight. Poor Simon was committed to the event, undeterred by a nasty cold. We completed our briefing and sorted the planned running order just as the first of the 500 guests started to trickle in.

The event progressed with a familiar cadence. Ball gowns and penguin suits leant an air of seriousness to proceedings, serious fun in honour of a serious challenge. The generosity of the large crowd was fuelled by the numerous guests whose lives have been touched by children with heart disease. There were many cheerful reunions celebrating friendships borne of mutual suffering. The mood and noise of the event typically built to a crescendo as the flow of champagne was accompanied by hot competition for auction prizes and the dazzling athleticism of the floor show. In keeping with a tradition of the event, the crowd was at some point brought to focus by a slide show. Families had sent in numerous 'before' and 'after' photos of their Heart Kids. Many of these photo couplets, like Malachy's, show at first a baby bloated and blue, covered in drains, dressings and medical tape. Many showed a blood-soaked surgical wound or a huge adult hand reaching into view, hoping to provide comfort. The second photo is more typically a beaming happy child, months or years later. Over and over the big screen depicts the apparent miracle by which the earlier chaos and crisis produces a happy thriving infant or teenager. Many of the images that night produced squeals of delight as the growing children defied the confronting reminders of how it all began.

Simon Reeve invited Malachy and me to step onto the stage in the chastened post-slide-show atmosphere. It was a chance for all to hear what it means to be a Heart Kid, from the mouth of the real thing, 12-year-old Malachy Frawley.

Stepping onto the stage that night was not just a young boy who had survived all the harrowing medical threats of his malformed heart, but also a boy who by now understood what it meant to be different. More than that, Malachy sensed that his disability had matured him in very particular ways. Underneath his strong considered manner was the weak vulnerable child who had more than once been teased at the local pool for wearing purple lipstick. He had brushed aside this charge by mumbling that he'd 'just been eating mulberries'. He was a boy who'd wrestled with one of the great 'What Ifs?'—'What if I'd been born with a healthy heart?'—and whose parents had often woken with the thought, 'What if they'd seen it on that very first ultrasound? What if they'd known what was coming and treated him before he 'crashed'? What if he'd had the right antibiotic a day earlier and it had saved his bowel?'

Malachy by now had good reason to feel content with his lot. He had been to Teen Camp and could now count other children like him amongst his friends. He had acquired and nurtured a lovely core group of friends with whom he would progress into high school. Maggie and I felt there were much worse things that could befall a family. We felt lucky to have this luminous presence in our life, with his spirit of resolve and self-possession, in spite of what could be seen as a lifetime of missing out. We counted the blessings of Mac's intellectual prowess and emotional adaptability, his happiness simply to be himself with all the limitations that entailed.

This package of qualities was unknown to his audience of five to six hundred people. They were willing this plucky little Heart Kid to deliver a poignant hiatus in the midst of the celebration. The audience watched politely, subdued, while Simon walked Malachy and me through a potted biography. Simon asked questions and Malachy replied to the limit of his knowledge, with me as back-up to fill in the gaps. Mac was resplendent in his dark suit, tie loosened in casual fashion as he poised on a bar stool at centre stage, Simon Reeve to his right, and his look-alike dad to his left. Mac seemed fully at home, at times working the crowd like a seasoned raconteur. We covered tales of his day one helicopter ride, his series of operations, his discovery of a sense of identity with his Heart Kid peers, his struggles to participate in ordinary childhood activities, and his appreciation of the efforts of HeartKids. He spoke of the gift of mobility that came with the Segway.

The interview turned to the more difficult area of the future. What Malachy's hopes and aspirations might be, and what we could hope for in the way of medical or surgical remedy. I explained for the gathering that Malachy's situation left him a little stranded, with poor exertional tolerance, but not necessarily much scope to improve things by drugs or operations. Another growth spurt had raised the question whether to undertake yet another operation to improve Malachy's oxygenation. This drew further questions from Simon.

Trying to do a Fontan procedure had been considered and debated. In short, a Fontan was major surgery. It would involve cutting off the major veins where they return to the heart and diverting them instead straight into the lungs.

It was subject to debate between his doctors, as well as at home, because Malachy's surgeon warned that surgery carried an increased immediate risk, that of dying from operative complications. He argued that doing nothing carried potentially the same long-term outcome, but with a more predictable decline at a later date. Also, some of Malachy's earlier 'What Ifs' had left him with complications that could hamper the proposed surgery. Mac's cardiologist on the other hand favoured proceeding, believing the altered circulation would put less strain on Malachy's heart than the current arrangement.

For the audience at the ball, I described my impression that Malachy was in a stable condition, and that Maggie and I hoped by the time surgery was necessary Malachy himself would be mature enough to play a major role in deciding whether to proceed.

At this point Simon redirected the questioning to Malachy.

Simon Reeve: 'Malachy, your thoughts on this?'

Malachy: 'If it gets to the stage where I really need it, haha, YES, but for now I'm just practically like a normal kid. So, I don't feel I need it, and I don't really want it. Um, 'cause it's pretty scary and also...' here he paused briefly lending weight to what followed. Malachy sat higher on the stool and spoke firmly, 'I'm proud of being blue'.

A communal hush and an intake of breath gave way to enthusiastic applause. I felt every parent in the room like me, would long to hear their child emulate that message: 'Mum, Dad, I'm proud to be ME'.

Malachy's reframing of his malformed self as a source of pride would define the young man that emerged into high school the following year. His personal resourcefulness imbued me with a deep confidence that he was equipped to cope with the cruel barbs of fate.

Simon repeated Malachy's statement for the audience, enjoying the defiant spark of his interview subject, before he concluded the Q & A.

Simon echoed what many in the audience must also have thought: 'Malachy, you're a fine young man. You'll be a Michael Parkinson before you know it.'

32

WRITINGS

Your memory is a monster; you forget — it doesn't. It simply files things away. It keeps things for you, or hides things from you — and summons them to your recall with a will of its own. You think you have a memory; but it has you!

— John Irving

At home the epic sagas Mac created for his figurines and stuffed toys could play out over days or weeks, then disappear without a trace when we made him tidy his room. His fertile mind generated an endless cycle of ephemeral marvels, here today and gone tomorrow. He was like a wasteful artist, refining his craft, casting one crumpled gem after another into recycling.

With advancing age, he kept all manner of journals, mainly to capture ideas that would otherwise pass through and disappear. He wrote and rewrote stories always wanting the next version to surpass its predecessor. The pages reflect his creativity, his perspicacity, his humour, his concerns and preoccupations, and not unexpectedly, hidden threads of autobiography.

Mac loved to share his vision for each new work. He loved to workshop ideas, and to entertain others with selected readings as he went along. Malachy had a particular way of casting his ideas before me. I was not always sure when he was soliciting criticism, and when he was intent on a display of incontestable brilliance. It forced me to walk a metaphorical tightrope, teetering between flattery and critique. If I misread his mood, Mac didn't make me pay too high a price. If I insulted him, he merely rejected my advice, especially if it threatened to dampen the narrative thrust. When he could see he'd sparked my admiration he would spin off more ideas with enthusiasm.

I loved to go on the dizzy ride of Malachy's adventure narratives in which events will usually be introduced at a drifting, leisurely pace, until at some point they accelerate dramatically with action and repartee piling on top of and across each other. Superhero asides and bad guy jibes compete with florid action sequences in a great adrenaline rush. Seemingly entire movie scenes spring from a single page of written text. Woah, slow down there, mate!

Songwriting had bursts of attention in Malachy's writing. Social themes are prominent in his lyrics, including expressions of concern for issues of equity, gender wars and race relations. These topics are interspersed with balancing tales of teen angst or indie rock love songs: complex romances with our hero plagued by self-doubt. He and his friends bandied around numerous names for their planned indie rock group, without ever making a firm choice. The vision was for a band ambitious to put potent issues before their adoring fans.

Max Martly was a theme Mac returned to, enriching the story with time. He remained adamant that the story had escaped his creative control somewhere between conception and its presentation on the silver screen. In defending myself I could never convince Mac of any value in my editing.

Mac and I discussed magical worlds. He assayed their various features in his imagination, including how these worlds would be entered and left, and how they would differ from our own world. Along the way, he conceived of various magical vehicles, with my favourite being his flying boats. He gave me a long, enthusiastic discourse on the features and narrative possibilities of pirate ships unbound by the limitations of lakes or oceans.

One element Malachy sought to bring to his 'other world' was the possibility of transformation as you pass from this world to the other. The constraints and limitations we as people suffer on earth are turned to our advantage on passing through. Perhaps this was akin to Harry Potter's transformation from orphaned loner to hero and saviour by the simple act of turning eleven. Malachy floated in the idea of a world populated by ethereal minion armies. In that world the size of your army was proportionate to your sufferings on this mortal plane. It is hard to avoid seeing that Malachy himself would be tremendously rewarded in an after-life governed by that rule. Every struggle brings more power and influence in the parallel universe, like a fantasy fiction version of Karma. Through his own struggles Mac found the idea of Karma attractive. Perhaps building on the success of his novels Mac could go on to start a new religion?

As the focus and desire to be a writer became clearer, one gift Malachy received along the way was a book called, *Rip the Page,* subtitled, *Adventures in Creative Writing.* It contained a wonderful variety of encouragements and stimuli to an aspiring author. Mac undertook the suggested exercises with earnestness. The effort he put into *Rip the Page* was far in excess of that applied to his schoolwork. There is a touching innocence to the way he obeys the author's instructions within the book's self-directed exercises.

One exercise invited Malachy to disclose six things he'd never told anyone. He wrote: *I've never told anyone that I'm scared of operations but love having scars and already have 11.*

On one page Malachy documented the priorities he adhered to. In the face of all he had suffered, Mac recorded a list of things he 'thanks his lucky stars for'. In order, spaced across the page he wrote:

My Friends	*My Family*	*HeartKids*
Segway	*Pens*	*My Brain*
Life in General		

33

VIETNAM

The most beautiful people we have known are those who have known defeat, known suffering, known struggle, known loss, and have found their way of out the depths.

— Elisabeth Kübler-Ross

Malachy woke to the puttering sound of a small engine after a night of gentle rocking on the calm waters of Ha Long Bay. Out the window was a dense mist, shrouding the spectacular limestone islands that thrust up through the deep green waters of coastal Vietnam. His excitement was hard to conceal as another day dawned in an exotic country where you get to eat noodles for breakfast. Even better, he had spent the night on a junk after a day adventuring through caves and waterways with his sister and some of his oldest friends, the twins Audrey and Charlotte (of *Max Martly* fame). A faint smell of curry and breakfast noodles helped him greet the day, as the salt-laden sea air enveloped him in comfortable warmth for a January day north of the equator.

This day in early 2012 could only get better, with pho on the menu, and an itinerary planning to take us past the famous 'fighting cocks', a pair of islands that seem to peck at each other like combative roosters when approached from the requisite angle. Already the Vietnam adventure had delivered in spades for Malachy, long a lover of Asian food and a devotee of cross-cultural understanding. Now just shy of his thirteenth birthday, this was Mac's first chance to experience the developing world, or what may be better called the majority world. UNICEF's beautiful publication *Children Just Like Me,* which gathers photos and stories from 11-year-olds the world over, had fascinated all of our children. The book had helped inspire in Mac the ambition to travel, and to melt away the false boundaries of nationality. It shows photographs of the children, often in traditional costumes, but also in their day-to-day life. There is a family photo for each, an image of their home and school, and pictures of their day's ration of food, and perhaps a favourite toy or hobby. Malachy had read with keen interest of Thi Lien, from the Dao hill tribe in Vietnam, who is pictured in the beautiful batik traditional clothes of her ethnic minority group. Sure enough, there was a picture of a bowl of pho, complete with chicken, vegetables and noodles. 'What a lucky kid!' he must have thought.

It was something of a family joke when anyone would grumble about anything. I would refer them back to *Children Just Like Me* with reference to the Thai boy Suchart who, we are informed, is 12 and lives in a temple called Wat Tanot, in the city of Ayuthaya. He is pictured in the saffron robes of a Buddhist monk, beaming the most serene of smiles back at the camera. Beside his portrait is another image, of Suchart sitting in his home. The home is a tin hut on stilts, with a woven roof seemingly made of reeds. There is a single shelf with one or two books and a candle. Suchart sits on a grass mat, which is the only bedding visible. Completing his worldly possessions is a small towel hanging on a wire. With masterful understatement we are told: *Thailand is a hot country and Suchart keeps his hut cool by propping open the door with bamboo sticks.* I shared with the children the first time we read this page, complete astonishment at the privations of this child's life. Further to that, we all agreed how truly, plainly happy the child appeared, unguardedly grinning at us off the page.

'Look at Suchart!' I exclaimed. 'He owns almost nothing and yet, he's still happy.'

Whenever any of us grumbled about our lot in the salubrious comfort of Nowra, on the wealthy eastern fringe of affluent Australia, there was a good chance someone would chip in with, 'Come on, Seamus, (or insert name!) remember Suchart? He has nothing—'

'BUT HE'S STILL HAPPY!' would come the chorus of response.

Malachy was loving his first chance to see, experience and test this phenomenon, of the contentment of the impoverished. Burning in him was the desire to experience that sense of joy that comes from within, to learn the secret of non-material ease. Every post was a winner from the time we landed.

Our first stop was in the seaside haven of Hoi An, where our town tour gave Malachy the royal treatment in the form of a cyclo. His own personal rider pedalled him through the hectic market stalls, bustling lanes of commerce and ancient historic buildings. All the while sounds and smells of the mysterious land wafted by. The colours of countless clothing stalls, paper lanterns, restaurants, tailors and shoemakers also assaulted his senses as he effortlessly wheeled his way along.

Hectic as Hoi An was, Malachy couldn't have guessed this was but a gentle introduction by comparison with the teeming mass of humanity he would encounter in the living, swarming city of Hanoi. Our base in the Old Quarter was heaven on earth, barring some challenges, for our young hero. Pho abounded at street stalls and shopfronts, along with all manner of treats, thrust our way by hawkers who crowded every inch of path and road. Any clothing, or toy or video or gadget a boy could imagine was on sale for a fraction of the price back home. Even better, they could all be haggled for, an unfamiliar challenge that immediately caught his fancy. Malachy had a clear sense of style emerging and took advantage of this environment to find a few items of clothing to fit the desired mould. The difficulty of having to make your way on foot through this mass of hawking, chattering, charming humans nearly undid Malachy, who at one point slumped exhausted on a gutter, just tens of metres from our destination. His father was apparently too caught up in the thrilling atmosphere to note Mac's slowing pace and increasingly heavy-panting breath.

Adding to Malachy's enjoyment, he'd taken an instant liking to our friend and guide, Hai, who had met us at the airport and regaled us with his tales of travel adventure, his keen wit and gentle mentoring manner. Hai was scrupulous in tending to Malachy's needs and easing the physical burden of mobility, with all manner of negotiated vehicular aids.

The world was growing before Malachy's eyes, and he was loving it.

All of this fed into the mix as Malachy ascended to the top deck of our junk on that misty morning in Ha Long Bay. The world was vast and was his oyster. He was loved by family and friends and strangers were easily enough engaged. Food, while a necessity, was proving a source of immense pleasure. The tools to build his personal style were accessible at his whim. The future held only ever more of these joys and consolations.

I raised my camera to capture the mood of the moment, as the fighting cocks moved into view ahead. Malachy turned to the camera, serenity beamed from his face. The eyes stared deep into the camera, as if steeled to embrace an expansive future. All that will be is held captive in those brown eyes. His hair is tousled by the light breeze, wisps of it heading this way and that, while a quiff heads backwards in the direction of the paired mystical islands in the background. Wearing the comfort of his favourite hoodie, his lips curl into a smile, with just a hint of mischief, but overwhelmingly stating to the world, much like Suchart, whatever has befallen me, 'I AM HAPPY'.

In this captured moment I see the boy who was unveiling the man who will be.

34

SOUNDTRACK OF YOUTH

To be honest, the problem with all the music being produced in England at the moment is it's boring Indie Shit.

— Noel Gallagher

Malachy toyed with the lukewarm water that half-filled the bathroom sink. There was a slight smirk and a nervous edge to his posturing as I approached from the lounge room, reaching for the can of shaving foam as I entered. Maggie and I had noticed the darkening of Malachy's upper lip, as his moustache began to deepen in colour and grow to be a noticeable sign of emerging adulthood. We were determined he wouldn't be one of those boys whose adolescence brings the semblance of neglect, where no one bites the bullet to advise, 'Son, it's time you learnt to shave'.

We had recently returned from Vietnam and Mac's thirteenth birthday was approaching. Physically he was less diminutive, showing signs of inheriting my height. This suggested his short stature was a matter of growth delay, related to his chronic illness rather than a lack of tallness genes.

Mac removed his shirt for the inaugural shaving ritual. His upper body was spare-shouldered and slender, bearing the scars of his many surgical interventions. No part of him was very muscular, though what muscle he had on his abdomen was easily defined, amongst further scars, in the virtual absence of a fat layer. Mac's legs were stick-like, as he'd never had the endurance to give them much work. This was amplified by the impairment of circulation through his right femoral artery, whose collateral vessels never grew to match those in the neighbouring leg.

Many of the elements which would define the teenaged Malachy had solidified into place by this time. He had an entrenched love of what he liked to refer to as 'British Post Punk Revival Indie Rock'—as the UK became the epicentre of his preferred bands. He spent hours listening to the lilting, sometimes convoluted lyrics of his favourite bands, even formulating a list of those he considered the greatest of all time. This list was headed by the much-loved Arctic Monkeys, who pushed every button for Malachy with their fusion of snappy, clever understated lyrics, with what Rick Martin from NME labelled, 'their brilliant post-garage melodic racket', somewhat presciently as their first album awaited release in 2005. Less obvious choices included Tokyo Police Club, a band who I remember once prompted Malachy to ask me, 'Why is it that Indie bands have such great lyrics?' Mac's list also honoured The Libertines, Modest Mouse, and The Vaccines. The Wombats went in and out of favour, as their more 'pop' sound mingled with verbal gems that set Malachy thinking, such as their description of a lucky break with accommodation. Their song *Jump into the Fog* had impressed Malachy with the way meaning emerged from the apparently simple lyrics. After, 'What a great achievement it was, to get a hotel room this late', he'd enjoyed the dawning moment when they moved on to, 'I bet they charge by the hour here', as he realised the implications of such a short rental period.

These and other similar bands and songs were the soundtrack of the period that found he and I poised before the mirror for what would be Malachy's first shave. I explained some of the detail.

'So, Mac, first you have to wet your skin.' He splashed tentatively from the basin.

'Then get a bit of shaving cream on your hands.' I squirted a blob of the minutely bubbled foam onto my own hand, touching some to the tip of his nose, then handed him the can. Timidly he depressed the nozzle which, with a gurgling noise, spat out a dribble of white pasty soap.

'Harder, Mac,' I entreated, before wishing I'd curbed my enthusiasm, as a mushroom cloud of foam billowed out of his waiting left hand. He chuckled with delight as the foam broke free and he madly dabbed it at me and a passing sibling. A foam fight beckoned as I wrested back control of the situation with some barked instructions.

This period in his life was also a time of new alliances, as Malachy found he could detect like-mindedness in those he encountered. This included one fertile long weekend with family friends, which morphed into a writers' retreat for the next great indie band, whose potential names were debated at length by the shores of Jervis Bay. The members, Mac.F, Soph, and The Willster projected a future in which 'The Procrastinators', or more favoured 'The Prophets' would regale audiences with their driving barrage of sound and incisive lyrical offerings. They churned out the lyrics and mapped the intended sound for some 20 tunes, which they gathered in a blue A4 folder, earmarked for further development. That folder encapsulates the angst of the era, with objections to bullying, tales of rejection and love unrequited, and the sweet victory of justice over popular acclaim.

There is the straining sadness of *I Have a Heart*, which includes the lyrics:

> I have a heart, I have a heart.
> You don't put yours to good use.

Bemoaning the limitations of his own malformed body. Or the line in the sand, drawn against the sheep-like adherence to mainstream pop culture:

> You always think about what you wear
> When I get ready without a care.
> You have a professional do your hair

> It's the best and anywhere
> else; you never bin there.

One song, *Recollections*, explores the gap between the pictorial record and the lived reality of an occasion:

> They're not an accurate recollection of the times,
> 'cause you're always asked to smile
> Or say CHEESE.
> It makes you always look happy,
> OH, PLEASE.

The chuckling boy with the furry upper lip gave no outward hint of complex thoughts and emotions that swirled in the vault of his skull, finding voice amongst his friends, and given form in that blue A4 ring-binder. His playful antics gave no hint of the inner reflective life that would lead him to announce a choice of song for his own, unplanned, funeral. For the record, the choice was *Float On* by Modest Mouse, chosen for the prominent sentiment that life should not be spent worrying about what might have been. 'We'll all float on OK', is the song's repeated refrain ordained by Malachy as his personal commemoration. Strange as it may seem, it wasn't completely foreign to our children to anticipate their own remembrance, as Niamh had long before taken dibs on Coldplay's *Fix You* whose refrain, 'Tears stream, down your face, when you lose something you cannot replace', leaves little wriggle room to escape the cause of your intense sadness.

After an amiable struggle, this boy whose hidden life included writings about teenage angst, vague anticipation of his own demise, and yearnings for fairness in the world, stood before the mirror, razor poised to carve its way through a smooth white beard of foam.

Malachy had a way of bringing a sense of moment to the simplest things. On the cusp of removing his first set of facial bristles, with a flourish of his razor, he paused.

'Dad, you know what this means, don't you?' He grinned in my direction.

'No, Mac, what?'

'D-Money, this means I'm a man now.'

35

MULTIMEDIA MAN EMERGES

To be nobody but yourself in a world which is doing its best night and day to make you like everybody else means to fight the hardest battle which any human being can fight and never stop fighting.

— E.E. Cummings

Malachy had long understood he could play a role in inspiring other children by modelling a successful adjustment to his lot in life. Malachy started high school in 2012. It was a time of social expansion. He started to realise that he had stared down challenges beyond the understanding of most children his age. The weakness of his body taught him to take nothing for granted and forced him to develop resilience in the face of repeated failure and exclusion. He became adept at spotting his own failings and making light of them. He started to mix his prescient understanding of life with self-deprecating humour and acquired new friends readily.

YouTube was part of the zeitgeist, and Malachy loved watching young stars of the internet's short-blog format. The celebrities he most appreciated were the producers of funny memes laughing at themselves. His forays into public disguises such as 'Jarred' came to be seen as practise runs. Malachy invented an array of alter egos for his own YouTube channel, and stepped onto the stage through short funny posts. His personal channel was named after the character who first took him to the silver screen, Max Martly.

In a skit entitled, *Earl Grey Incident*, Malachy sits at his drum and confidently eyes the camera. Behind him is his much-loved indie band wall of fame. With his tie secured in a Windsor knot, Malachy affects a casually intimate tone as he raises his brow in reminiscence, being the amiable raconteur, lulling the viewer into a shared confidence. With a hint of absurdity his camera cuts to a shoe on the ground, then the broken zipper of his jacket. He is showing mundane inadequacies of his daily grind. There are more quirky cuts, a disappearing shirt, tie changes and some character costuming as the story progresses. Malachy narrates a calamitous morning of taking himself off to school. He bumbles his way out the door, dishevelled and dreary, feeling uncool and vulnerable, into the walking path of a men's drug rehabilitation group. Mac parodies the men in character. At one point he makes a conspiratorial lean into the camera to show off the tattoo work on his forearms, dropping asides about his talent for body art. The skit ends just as Mac is opening his front gate, trying to look cool for the rehab crowd. His mother pops up and babies him with instructions for the day ahead. His virile image is skewered at the critical point in time, as the one-time junkies are streaming past.

Earl Grey Incident had me laughing right through, feeling yet more love and admiration for the man emerging in Malachy. It is so well composed, and confidently styled, I felt there was a real possibility there was a star being born in our house. Regardless of that, Mac was having great fun, and acquiring new skills. Feeling cautious about the brave new world of self-publication on social media, I was also relieved that his vignette was suitably anonymous. As his YouTube catalogue grew there were other funny skits listing his life's 'fails', a rant about issues of gender equity, and a mock celebration on reaching the milestone of three subscribers.

Maggie and I had cautioned against open use of his own identity on the internet, to protect Mac's privacy, and the true identity of his characters. Mac relished the privacy challenge and found ways to reference real events and places while covering his tracks with panache. Always clever and passionate, Mac veered into politics and culture wars. I showed some parental hypocrisy; having spent years aiding and abetting Malachy's fearlessness in the clash of ideas, I once crossed the line from mentor to censor. 'Malachy,' I said, and I cringe to recall it, 'it's great that you want to speak about the injustices boys suffer in the name of equality, but I'm just not sure the time is right to champion boys' rights. Remember girls have had it tough through history? You need to be a bit careful how people might interpret … etc.' He ignored me, stuck to his guns, and posted a mournful plea on behalf of the male children of Australia.

As Malachy's foray into social media progressed, our knowledge of him also grew. The insights he posted for the world at large had strong peer currency and cache. This allowed us to be party to the real culture of our teenager in a way that parents rarely are. As he revealed more to his viewers, we learned more of his humour and his concerns. More riveting than the content itself was the man we saw emerging. As a father, I had sweated on Malachy's every milestone from the minute of his birth. Maggie and I had first feared he would never see a birthday, then never attend school, then maybe not high school. Mac had never had an outlet for the stage presence and confident bearing that now silenced our doubts. A young man with swagger and poise had stepped in, replacing the protected, coddled baby I'd been so slow to let go of.

This emerging digital media man brought me inexplicable joy, symbolised in my mind by a magnificent butterfly breaking free of its chrysalis, or the ugly duckling's debut as a beauty. It was a wholly unexpected source of pleasure, of comfort, of confidence in the future.

Coinciding with this, other consolations were falling into place. Malachy's circle of friends expanded apace at school, and his range of activities blossomed as the bounds of the possible opened up. Like-mindedness began to influence his acquisition of new friends, as drama classes and drumming became valued hobbies. Even the bus trip to school became an avenue of growth as the daily commute brought new alliances, including a budding friendship with 'the girl on the bus'.

Mystery attached to Mac's particular friend and confidante from the morning bus route, not because he hid anything or disguised any affection he might feel, but because this was beyond our parental reach. The children preferred the long bus route to school, despite the fact Maggie taught at St John's, and could drive them there in a fraction of the time. The bus was their secret life, where we knew none of the players. By small town coincidence 'the girl', Camille, was the daughter of a woman I knew. The mother surprised me one day by telling me of an extensive flow of text messages between our two households. The bus route through Nowra had brought together two compatible, original young minds.

Lucky kids. Lucky parents. Our child whom we'd always known as the most lovable of people we felt sure was now being found lovable by the world at large.

All the ingredients of future happiness were gathered. The family set sail to steady the passage through Mac's teenage years, glad of the type of adult we saw evolving before our eyes. As with any child we had no idea what adventures lay ahead, but we dared to feel excited by the promise of the chapters to come. Maggie and I pictured Malachy as the youth of 18, the man of 30, and beyond to a point. Naturally, there was less certainty the further ahead we dreamed.

If I'd thought of it then I may have said to Malachy, 'Raconteur, author, comedian, drummer, film director, Heart Kid, tie-wearing son, brother and friend: the future is yours'.

36

PLANS AND IDEAS

We should aim for our children to be good people, and to live ethical lives that manifest concern for others as well as for themselves.

— Peter Singer

Malachy's precocious interest in meaning and purpose made the great ethical question, 'How should I live?' an occasional topic of discussion. His older siblings were in the process of selecting the possible direction of their university careers through 2013. Niamh was choosing her senior years' school subjects, while Seamus was sitting the final school examinations, and Imogen looking at repurposing her mathematics degree towards engineering.

The moral universe Malachy wrestled with had three main types of idea in competition. Each had a different claim on his emerging adult consciousness and conscience.

First in line was the availability of a god, with a codified set of rules to live by. Mac had been taught the religious framework of the Catholic Church. Thirteen years of practice and teachings, along with almost nine years in Catholic schools, both in Australia and Ireland, helped Malachy feel confident in the Catholic process of ethical decision-making.

Mac was also aware of the more intuitive appeal to reason exemplified by a utilitarian understanding, which was more akin to the dominant secular thinking of the time. I had been influenced by the utilitarian philosophers John Stuart Mill and Jeremy Bentham, and occasionally mentioned their guiding principle at the dinner table: The greatest happiness of the greatest number is the foundation of morals and legislation.

Thirdly, Malachy had exposure to existentialist ideas, which were also raised at our dinner table, with Imogen having taken great pleasure in the discovery of Jean-Paul Sartre. Existentialism had great appeal as a novel set of ideas, but it wasn't helpful for Malachy who ran the risk of falling into the inevitable trap of existential angst. Angst is the feeling of despair people experience when they are confronted by the absence of meaning in their life. It can make it hard to keep struggling on. Imogen reflected with good humour on the dark pleasure of existentialist thought with the tongue-in-cheek question, 'Why did I have to discover Existentialism now, when I'm so young? Life is supposed to have a meaning when you're only 20.'

For Malachy philosophical musings needed to be more than a fun thought exercise. Thinking was always more satisfying when he could apply it to something real.

The Catholic moral teachings about social justice made a lot of sense to Malachy. He enjoyed talking about some of those ideas with a local priest, Father Duane, whose parish youth group Malachy took part in. The unfairness of poverty was a recurring interest, particularly after he had seen how poverty played out in Vietnam.

Malachy also demonstrated a feel for utilitarianism. The theory was dwelt on by Malachy in discussions about the desirability of talents being shared out fairly amongst his group of friends. Vegetarianism and animal rights were also on the ethical radar of our children. Support for this came from vegetarians in the extended family, but also from the ideas of an Australian utilitarian philosopher, Peter Singer.

As Malachy took his first tentative steps into adult life, he and his parents had to work through some parallel dilemmas. Sometimes I would watch Malachy as he interacted with his friends or family, or engage in activities, and find my thoughts transported. Was he happy? Would he be happier if he could walk further and do more? Should he try for a heart transplant?

Uncertainty about this big question nagged away in the background. It was still possible that a successful transplant would help him walk further, but at the cost of heavy suppression of his immune system. Heart transplant would buy Malachy just a 50 percent chance of living another ten years, to age 23. The immune suppression would increase his risk of dangerous infections and of premature development of various cancers. Malachy had cheerfully adapted to his current activity level, but what if an operation could take him onto the greener grass of being more able? Where was the 'greater good' in this? I wondered whether Malachy could continue to be happy with a cautious, Buddhist style path, as John Stuart Mill once described: 'I have learned to seek my happiness by limiting my desires, rather than in attempting to satisfy them'.

In reality, a heart transplant was not on the cards. The most likely next step if the need for surgery arose was a Glenn shunt operation, the first step towards a Fontan type circulation. My daydreams often included wondering how long it might be before something happened to demand another round of surgery. It was more than mere daydreaming, because it was a recurring question. We knew Mac was proud of being blue, but how much limitation could he tolerate?

For his part, Malachy was working through questions about his own aspirations. I watched him give up on the unlikely dream of managing any modicum of sporting ability and bend more towards the life of the mind. Increasingly his choices of activity reflected his thinking that if he wanted to be a 'Child Prodigy', as an author, he had no time to lose. Why waste his time on the diverse activities of 'normal' adolescence? Why waste time on unnecessary learning, such as mathematics or science? Why plan for a future that is so riddled with uncertainty?

I had to pause and consider my thoughts one day when Malachy posed the question: 'Dad, how long do you think I will live?'

Calmly and slowly, wanting any tightness I felt to pass undetected in my tone, I replied: 'Mac, I don't know, but I hope it's well into adult life. Long enough, I hope, to take advantage of some new technology for your heart.'

'I feel pretty good now, Dad. If I can stay the way I am, that's okay by me.'

'Well, that's good, Mac. You know Dr Nunn thinks you can stay pretty stable like this for a long time.'

'Well, D-Money, I think that's what I'd like to do. I don't really want to do an operation if I don't have to. What I really want to do is write stuff, and I can do that pretty well now. I can put up with getting out of breath.'

I admired his clarity.

Maggie and I had chosen to send Seamus to boarding school for his senior years, and hope Malachy's illness wouldn't prevent him from having the same opportunity. Mac would get an excellent education, and a well-rounded school experience if he stayed in Nowra, but we didn't want heart disease to rob him of what we saw as a broadening and maturing experience. At the same time, Malachy gave no indication he would resent a 'lost opportunity', and pre-empted some of the deliberation about his schooling.

'D-Money, it costs a lot to go to boarding school, right? But the kids have to pay for their own university degrees? I know I want to go to university, so if I decide not to go to boarding school, would you pay for me to go to uni?'

'I guess so, Mac. Boarding school is pretty good, though. They're way into drama at the school. Every year level puts on an annual play. You'd have a play you could go to in every year up there. Also, did you see that thing in the newsletter about the boy in Year 9 who had his book published? You might find there's a whole bunch of writers you can link in with up there.'

'Yeah, I saw that, but Dad, I can write just sitting in my room. I don't really need to go to Sydney for that, and I've got a really cool bunch of friends in Nowra. I'm really happy with my friends. I think you'd be better off saving up for me to go to uni. Besides, you might be pretty worried about me up at school in Sydney.'

Mac was right about that. Maggie and I were both dreading the long-distance worry we knew lay ahead. We dreaded our powerlessness at the end of the phone line if something should go wrong with Malachy up in Sydney. I think Malachy was declaring his utilitarian hand. The greater happiness might well consist of keeping our baby close. If we were worried what he may miss out on by staying in Nowra, he wasn't.

Mac sketched out a basic plan of life. Write, and keep writing, until the magnum opus of Child Prodigiousness is complete. Stay in the safety of Nowra, enjoying the fun and energy of my friends, and the adoration of my parents. Keep polishing my ideas and my talents until they gleam with perfection. Then, once school is completed, onwards and upwards to the wider world, fountain pen in hand, the first of my publications tucked under my arm, and a colourful tie flapping over my shoulder.

Malachy, the author of the future, exuded such a confident sense of direction that nothing, it seemed, would stand in the way of his destiny.

Sartre's angst must defer to our future ambitions. A plan for the future takes little account of whether or not that future exists.

37

DRUM ROLL

He's got rhythm in his hands as he's tappin' on the cans.
— from *Gold* by John Stewart

I remember my first trip to the circus, when I was four years old. It was the very first time I heard drums used to build expectation of a drama to follow. The drums that day were warning of the dangers faced by a troupe of trapeze artists, and I recall being swept along in the building tension of the drums, culminating in a triumphant clashing of cymbals with every safe aerial catch.

The link between rumbling noises and expected drama has struck me as fascinating ever since.

Learning the drums seemed a natural fit with Malachy's emerging identity, partly because he was always drumming his domed fingers on every surface he encountered, but also because a rumbling voice inside me was forever hinting at possible drama to come.

Mac's traumatic beginnings ensured we were never fully free of worry for our fourth child. With Malachy, as with the circus, if there was the risk of drama, there was also vivid display, excitement and entertainment along the way. There was the expectant buzz of not knowing what was around the corner. Malachy showed a dramatic flair in the building of his identity, somehow believing or knowing his life had an audience. He bore the charisma of certainty that when he sought to engage you with a story of interest, you would find it as compelling as he intended.

Drum lessons were part of Malachy's emergence from the intense challenges of his life to that point. The prelude had been first survival, then endless wrestles with disability, and now the punchline was the fast-maturing Malachy we would come to know. High school became a fecund period, with Malachy leaping up with a 'Ta-Daa' to indicate the period of suspense was over. He seemed hungry to enjoy every new turn, as if to signify repeatedly, 'I've been waiting for this moment'.

The experimental threads of the identity Malachy wove were numerous as he tried out drama classes, writing, filming, activism and 'you-tubing'. Each activity brought new friends, as Malachy flushed out the good in the people he met, enthusing about their different qualities.

Happily for me, Malachy loved to share his thoughts about the events of the day.

'Oh, Dad, I got in this sort of argument on the bus.'

'Really, what happened?'

'Well, you know how there's all these guys from the Christian school on the bus? Well, I was asking them about Creation and the Big Bang.'

'Oh, yeah.'

'Yeah. And it doesn't make any sense. They believe God just made everything in seven days. So I asked them about the dinosaurs...'

Off it went from there. I felt a bit nervous he'd become the leper of the bus trip, a Catholic believer in science in a hostile sea of literal biblical belief. It wasn't to be the case. He seemed to know how to push the buttons of dissent without destroying the bonhomie. We heard more, in snippets, of the fun crowd on the bus, with the many children of our local mayor, and a few others of particular interest.

Refreshingly, the bus, as with drama classes, had the benefit of taking Malachy outside the safe confines of his familiar school crowd. I would drive to collect him from drama classes and have to beckon him away from a cluster of three or four new people he'd found resonance with. As a fully-fledged teen, Malachy had to tread the line of not telling his parents too much, partly no doubt to avoid enquiry about potential love interests, but also to start feeling the freedom to develop away from the microscope of parental concern.

Malachy's contemplation of where his life to date had landed him brought a few things into clearer focus. He had firmed in his career ambition to be an author, as soon as possible.

He realised too, that he could be a leader amongst his peers. People looked to him for insight and initiative, having found him skilled in both departments.

Despite his famed blue pride, it also occurred to Malachy that his physical limitations were an impediment to his ambitions. He was growing tired of being tired. This led us to the long-deferred contemplation of corrective heart surgery.

Malachy's long-serving cardiologist, Stephen Cooper, favoured a surgical adjustment to his circulation, not foreseeing a dramatic increase in his abilities, but aiming for a more durable circulation, with less in the way of long-term complications. Maggie and I both felt very risk averse on Malachy's behalf, given how well-adjusted he had always appeared in the face of his impairment. Over-protectiveness of children is difficult enough to suppress in the era of helicopter parenting. This is much more so when that child's life has repeatedly been in the balance with every milestone so hard-won. Dr Cooper recommended we book a time to consult with the surgeon.

HeartKids Australia had once organised a consumers' conference about children's heart disease. Not a medical conference, but a conference to help and inform families like ours. One of the speakers was a young surgeon who contended that we don't need to protect our children as much as we do, even the ones with heart disease. Making his case, he showed video footage of a man called Shaun White, who is the most accomplished Olympic snowboarder of all time. The audience watched mesmerised as Shaun was dropped from a helicopter and tore away down an unmarked mountain performing stunts and avoiding rocks and other obstacles with consummate skill and absolute fearlessness. Parents of sick, cyanotic children were wowed by the footage of Shaun in a half-pipe, twirling through the air before skidding back down the hard icy tube. They were stunned when the doctor advised, 'Shaun White is a Heart Kid'.

Silence.

'Shaun White was born with Tetralogy of Fallot and had two open heart operations before the age of one.'

The term 'tetralogy' derives from the presence of four abnormalities in the heart of a child born with this problem. The effect of these is to make the child blue, like Malachy, and require corrective operations in early life. Tetralogy of Fallot produces a classical X-ray appearance of a boot-shaped heart. A likeness to the boot shape was the reason the paediatrician had suggested this diagnosis when Malachy became ill on his first day of life.

Shaun White has said of his heart disease: 'It instilled a bit of a fight in me from the get-go'.

Take home message: death-defying stunts no problem for Heart Kid.

So here I was, contemplating the over-protection of the species Heart Kid and, true to type, feeling fearful of the risks involved in possible heart surgery. All things considered, we bit the bullet and took Malachy to see the surgeon. Maggie and I needed to feel convinced it was the right thing and felt Malachy should also be allowed to weigh the risks and benefits for himself. Dr Nunn was no longer around, so we were referred to a new surgeon, Dr Chard in February 2013.

The interview to plan and consider the Glenn shunt operation was quite long. Our questions were answered in some detail, with plenty of food for thought. Malachy pursued his own line of consideration, wanting to hear of the likely improvement in his fitness. One of the key factors for Malachy was that he was needing more help moving around at school. He had good friends who were happy to walk with him, and often be late for class on his account. Sometimes he needed a piggy-back up a slope, which was a decisive factor in bringing him to the point of seeking a fix. He had wearied of the gentle uphill climb to K Block, which he could never reach without assistance. Mac was also interested to discuss the possibility of his finger clubbing diminishing. To make the best decision we also had to discuss the downside.

Maggie asked, 'So, Dr Chard, what complications should we be aware of?'

A range of potential technical failings to do with pressures and fluid build-up in the legs or lungs were canvassed along with the standard infection and bleeding type things we'd always been advised of. Serious complications such as stroke or heart injury were cited as possible.

Then this: 'An operation of this scale would carry with it a five to ten percent mortality, a five to ten percent chance of death during the operation'.

Maggie and I both felt Malachy stiffen. His bodied straightened just enough to be perceptible. His face dropped ever so slightly. The talk dried up. For two-and-a-half hours we drove the route home to Nowra, aware that Malachy was quiet, unlike himself. A light had dimmed.

The next day all seemed forgotten, Malachy's day-face was the same as ever. The chat was back, the news that Mac was having a date booked for surgery went out and we resumed our usual service. The admission for the Glenn shunt operation was arranged for the middle of March.

Malachy continued to look forward with all the enthusiasm we'd come to love. He hardly skipped a beat when the next, unexpected challenge popped up.

Maggie noticed Malachy's back had begun to look a bit asymmetrical, which led us down a path of investigation for scoliosis. Sure enough, his back was crooked, but not only that, one leg was shorter than the other. The blocked artery in his right leg had caught up with Mac. The reduced blood supply had stunted the growth on that side. There was another unexpected X-ray finding too, Malachy had an extra vertebral bone in his spine.

Would this be the last straw for Malachy? A world of resilience had built up around his heart disease, but now he had to add a crooked back and a gammy leg to his list of woes. It seemed to the family he had suffered enough without this. It made us want to scream, 'WHY MALACHY?' at the top of our lungs.

Maggie and I cried in private about the unfairness of it.

Malachy stayed cool.

The orthopaedic surgeon, Dr Gray, gathered all the evidence and concluded that both the spinal abnormality and the shortened leg shouldn't cause big problems. Malachy would need spinal X-rays and check-ups from time to time, monitoring the need for corrective surgery, but no immediate action. The heel of his shoe could be built up to lengthen his right leg.

38

DISCERNING THE SPIRITS

Several years have now elapsed since I first became aware that I had accepted, even from my youth, many false opinions for true.

— René Descartes

The secret of Malachy's equanimity in the face of challenge is hard to pinpoint. One simple explanation could be that he was the inheritor of 'The God of Good Outcomes' that had kept us hopeful through the starkest challenges of Malachy's early years. Malachy had probably not heard of this particular variation on the Almighty, but The GGO didn't spring from nowhere.

Maggie and I had engaged in spiritual seeking over many years. Our Catholic backgrounds had not exposed us to any scandalous abuses, so as young adults we felt safe in our practice of the Catholic faith. We had been part of a variety of prayer and meditation groups over many years, finding reflection and contemplation calming.

Meditation had made intuitive sense to me from my first exposure to it in my early teens. The Jesuits taught me meditation in my school years, following their model known as Ignatian spirituality. It involves a technique of contemplating your life in silent prayer, taking note of which thoughts make you feel happiest. The idea was to choose the path that would bring most happiness. To paraphrase poorly: Thoughts which lead to peace are Good. Those which leave you flat are Bad.

The ultimate goal of Ignatian spirituality was to achieve a peaceful state in which you felt so secure that you had the courage to live well, indifferent to the petty ups and downs of your daily existence, becoming neither derailed by hardship nor excessively inflated by good fortune. Whether by nature or nurture, apart from a brief period as Makatoa, Malachy had been a model of Ignatian indifference. He was a brave boy, and had remained positive despite his traumatic journey, and showed little interest in being buoyed by transient pleasures of materialism.

Ignatian ideas had also been influential in the Jesuit schooling of René Descartes, born in 1596, now hailed as the father of modern philosophy. Descartes' scepticism, or radical doubt, is encapsulated by the famous Latin statement: *Cogito ergo sum* (I think, therefore I am).

I had read a translation of Descartes' original essay setting out his reasoning. One day a conversation with my fourth child brought Descartes' essay to mind:

'Dad?' Mac's earnest tone captured my attention.

'Yes, Mac.'

'I've been thinking,' as he sought eye contact, briefly hesitant, 'I've been thinking: how do I know I'm not dreaming?'

My ears pricked. This had potential. 'Yes…'

'Well, I think I'm awake, but even when I have dreams, I think I'm awake. They seem real to me at the time. So, since this seems real, that means it could be a dream.'

'I like it, Mac.'

Warming to the task, I saw his brow furrow with intent: 'I thought I might prove I'm awake by pinching myself, but I can hurt myself in dreams anyway, so it doesn't really help. How do I even know if you are real, or if you are just my Dad in my dream?'

'Well, Mac, you're right, and I might be just sitting in this chair in my jeans, talking to you. Or I might be dreaming that I'm sitting in this chair. You're sounding like Descartes!'

This is what he was sounding like:

> How often have I dreamt that I was in these familiar circumstances, that I was dressed, and occupied this place by the fire, when I was lying undressed in bed?
>
> ...I perceive so clearly that there exist no certain marks by which the state of waking can ever be distinguished from sleep, that I feel greatly astonished; and in amazement I almost persuade myself that I am now dreaming.[10]

Later that night I joked to Maggie that I could have saved myself a lot of time, all the time I'd spent reading philosophy, if I'd known my own child was the reincarnated Father of Modern Philosophy.

Why indeed would a boy preoccupied with the nature of reality, the puzzle of existence, and becoming an author, concern himself with crooked backs, gammy legs, or imperfect hearts?

---

10 René Descartes, 1641. *Meditation 1.* 'Of the Things of Which We May Doubt'.

39

SCHOOLYARD ACTIVISM

I'm for truth, no matter who tells it. I'm for justice, no matter who it is for or against. I'm a human being, first and foremost, and as such I'm for whoever or whatever benefits humanity as a whole.

— Malcolm X

Malachy brought fun to most of his interactions, but also paradoxically there was a seriousness to his presence. He loved to laugh, but also to believe that things mattered. A hint of urgency attended his thinking, such that Mac seemed at times desperate for the world to improve before his eyes. Part of him always sensed that his actions needed to impress an audience, as if believing Milan Kundera's assertion that, '...we are only what other people consider us to be', yet he was often heedlessly engaged with the issues of the time. There was both an image to be tended and a legacy to be preserved. A version of Malachy who was charismatic and fun to be around, and the other one whose immortality needed guarding, whose reputation would outlive its owner.

The drive to bring issues to resolution was strong enough to carry with it some management headaches. Since primary school Malachy had been known to enter the political fray within the extended family. He was still only very young when he warmed to the challenge of debating his very conservative maternal grandfather. Understandably, given Malachy's tender age, Barry deemed him a mere mouthpiece of his father. To my chagrin I was forced to plead helplessness to control the flow of his ideas. Barry scoffed at my denial, leaving me to wear the blame for Malachy's left-leaning tendency.

Barry was an ardent supporter of the conservative side of politics, creating potential for uncomfortable dissent around the dinner table. The prime minister around the turn of the century, John Howard, was a master politician on the conservative side and a very divisive man. Mr Howard was loved by those who felt he stood up for their traditional values and universally loathed by those with progressive ideas. My parents-in-law were among his admirers.

Malachy was still in primary school on one occasion when Maggie's parents, Colleen and Barry, booked in for a short stay with us in Nowra. I was mindful of wanting to preserve harmony and keen not to mar the pleasure of their visit with any embarrassing political stand-off. Anticipating the risk, Maggie and I held a briefing.

At breakfast, with all the children present, we held an impromptu family meeting.

Maggie opened proceedings: 'Okay, children, Nanna and Parky are coming today for a bit of a stay'.

'Yeah, we know ... And?'

'AND, we want to enjoy their company, so it's important we don't talk about things that will get people upset.'

'Like what?' Malachy asked, as if he didn't know.

'Mac,' said Imogen, 'I think they mean *you*, not talking POLITICS'.

'Yes, Mac,' I intoned, in my best Calm Dad voice, 'we know you like discussing issues, but you can't change Parky and he just gets upset. It gets a bit uncomfortable, Mac, because he thinks we've put you up to it, and we DON'T WANT to get stuck talking about that stuff, OKAY? So, no politics and definitely don't mention John Howard. There's plenty of other stuff to talk about.'

'You guys get it, too,' added Maggie. 'We just don't need to get stuck on those things—we don't see much of my parents these days.'

'Yes, Mum,' came the chorus, and we dispersed to our different activities, with a final coercive glare at Malachy.

Late in the morning the doorbell rang. Bags were hauled from the car, and the grandparents shown into the kitchen. Nearly five hours of driving from Cootamundra to Nowra is no mean feat when you're eighty or so years old. The kettle squealed to announce its readiness and a welcoming ritual pot of tea was poured. The pleasant familiarity of family togetherness settled on the room, while we exchanged the usual greeting banter, confirmed that work was going well, everyone's health was good, and the children enjoying school.

As the standard greeting ran its course there was a slight lull, a void from which the next round of conversation would arise. I tilted my head to commence but was beaten to it. First off the mark into the restful moment sprang Malachy.

'So, Parky, I have to write something for school about a great person. Can you name someone you think is great?'

'Let me think about that, Malachy. What about Don Bradman?'

'Yeah, but what about living people? You know who I think is one of the greatest people alive?'

'No, Malachy, tell me.'

'Peter Garrett.'

(Pregnant pause)

Peter Garrett had long been a hit with Malachy, as the lead singer of Midnight Oil. Their explosive rock with a strong social conscience blared out of Malachy's room as much as any of his favourites, and for a time in his infancy had been the only music he listened to. So far so good! Somewhere along the way, by the time we sat down to our convivial cup of tea, the band had dissolved. Before their parting of ways, they had famously performed at the closing ceremony for the Sydney Olympic Games, in the year 2000. They had performed a protest song, *Beds Are Burning*, a song of yearning for the land rights of Australia's traditional indigenous owners, and symbolic reconciliation with their British and

European conquerors. John Howard was present in the official party at the ceremony. Mr Howard had previously declared *Beds Are Burning* his favourite Midnight Oil song. As Prime Minister he had earned some notoriety for his refusal to apologise to Indigenous Australians for their dispossession at the hands of the 'civilising' British and their Australian-born descendants. Much had been made of his apparent inability to utter, on behalf of the nation, the simple word, Sorry.

As they performed, with more than a billion people around the world watching the live telecast, The Oils peeled off their shirts to display another layer beneath with the word **SORRY** emblazoned clearly on each band member. It proved highly controversial. How dare they embarrass John Howard on the world stage? How dare they bring politics to the Olympics?

After the band dissolved, Peter Garrett made a successful transition into politics, starting as a Shadow Minister for Climate Change, fighting against the Howard Government, and ending up as the Minister for the Environment, Heritage and the Arts under Prime Minister Kevin Rudd. At the time of our quiet cup of tea, climate change—a pet topic of Malachy's—was a source of vigorous contention between the 'left' and 'right' of Australian politics.

(Pause over)

'Really, Malachy? Peter Garrett! Why?'

'Well, he's a great singer and he's a great fighter for the environment. He stands up for what he believes. And he's a really smart man.'

'I'm sorry to hear you say that, Malachy; I think he's a very misguided man. If you ask me, I'd say Mr Howard—he was a great leader.'

Niamh, eyes wide, discreetly shot an exasperated look at Malachy. Seamus studiously betrayed no emotion. In five minutes, we'd reached exactly where we had planned never to go.

'AND Peter Garrett's going to help us win the fight against global warming.'

'Oh, here we go now, global warming. Who's been telling you about global…'

Alas, too late, we found a way to eject the young protagonist from the room.

I groaned.

Malachy smiled.

*

Concern was etched on Malachy's face as he arrived home one Friday. It wasn't just the familiar weariness of the walk home. A worried frown told me something weighed on him. It crossed my mind that there'd been no bullying since he'd moved to high school. Was this the signal it had returned? A mild strain entered his tone.

'D-Money, why do people think they know better than the scientists? What do they base their opinions on?'

Relief walked hand in hand with amusement, as I pondered the curiousness of a 12-year-old who spent his days worrying about anthropogenic global warming. As much as we counselled him that his friends may see things differently as they get older, Malachy was not content to allow parental influence as an excuse for lazy conservatism. 'They're just reflecting their parents' views, Mac', was not a satisfactory response.

American neo-conservatism was a prevalent influence in Malachy's high school years, with a belligerent and obstructive Congress giving President Obama no respite. This helped encourage the Australian political discourse further to the right. Denial of the science behind global warming was a rallying cry which had shoe-horned Tony Abbott into leadership of the Liberal Party, and with that change it became the norm for socially conservative Australians to stop caring about scientific truth. The idea that a lie repeated often enough becomes truth to many people infuriated Malachy.

More than once our afternoon tea discussion revolved around conversational strategy. Malachy felt acutely the problem of having no starting point to a rational argument when the conservative position relied fundamentally on denial of facts. I felt his pain, but also thought it was worth letting him wrestle with that. I loved that the contest of ideas was interesting to Malachy.

While his debating skills were gradually honed during lunchtime impasses, Malachy was forced to recognise some arguments could not rise above the politics of the time. Fortunately, his sense of justice expanded to include areas other than the polarising litmus test of climate. He was prepared to chance his arm on any topic, without being mired in the rules of political correctness.

His reformist sympathies didn't stop him from venturing into hazardous territory when it came to gender politics. Malachy had filmed himself having a rant about his feeling that men and boys were given a hard time in the media, and in school disciplinary procedures. Clearly, he felt himself to be innocent of the crimes by which males have entrenched themselves in positions of power. He didn't hide his frustration at what he felt was an unfair public discourse about the negative qualities of men. I cringed a bit, knowing how readily the 'poor, maligned unlucky boys' line could be misinterpreted as ignorant or bigoted.

Refugees were frequently in the media as an issue, with arriving in Australia by boat being successfully portrayed as somehow immoral. The demonising of people seeking help in Australia bothered Malachy. His travel experience in Vietnam had exposed him to the majority world. What Malachy saw there gave him a strong sense of what good fortune he had to be born in Australia, and as a corollary of that he had seen for himself why people might want to join us. Vietnam, of course, is by no means as harsh or threatening as the conflict and domestic persecution many people are fleeing when they apply to Australia for asylum.

In a quiet moment, some months after returning from the Vietnam adventure, Malachy shared a reflection on the relative merits of the two countries.

'D-Money, I love Vietnam. If I lived there, I would have pho for breakfast every day. Wasn't the food delicious there?'

'It was great, wasn't it, Mac?'

'Yeah. Dad, but Dad, if we lived in Vietnam, they wouldn't have the kind of medical care I needed. I probably wouldn't be alive now, would I?'

'Probably not, Mac, I think in most parts of the world people with an abnormality like yours wouldn't make it out of hospital.'

'So, I'm only alive because I was born in Australia. That's not really fair, is it? But it's lucky for me. What if I was born ten years earlier?'

'Ten years, I think you would have been okay … but if you'd been born the same year as me, I don't think so.'

'I'm lucky to be alive.'

'Yeah.'

I don't know how I would live if I knew I owed my every breath to a trick of timing and geography. How Malachy would distil this insight in his attitude and actions was an intriguing question to observe. It forms part of the creative mystery of his identity. Combing through the evidence of his history suggests he knew his life was a gift. A gift not just for him to enjoy but bestowing on him a joy to be shared.

40

OPERATION TIME

Life shrinks or expands in proportion to one's courage.

— Anaïs Nin

The scent of disinfectant tinged the brightly lit sterility of the pre-operative ward at The Hospital for Children, Westmead. Staff of various types, their specific role designated by differing pyjama colours marched purposefully this way and that. The sound of trollies echoed around the barren cubicle where an emotional huddle supported Malachy to the cusp of a long-forestalled operation.

It had finally come to this: Imogen, Maggie and I clustered at the bedside, nerves jangling, a tear or two straining to slide down a cheek unnoticed, smiles of encouragement fixed in place.

Malachy wriggled in the bed as the anaesthetist and the anaesthetic nurse approached to go about their work. Frozen terror was not his style, so while some fear must have niggled at him, to all appearances he welcomed these experts as not only skilled technicians but as another audience for his humour.

The decision to be here, minutes away from the first incision of the bidirectional Glenn procedure, was not taken lightly nor quickly. This procedure would involve removing one of the routes by which blood returned to Malachy's heart, the superior vena cava, and diverting this return to feed directly into the lungs. The essential goal was to obviate the need to pump a large volume from the heart to the body and lungs with every beat, and instead have some of the blood return through the lungs, passively receiving oxygen en-route. Malachy had spent years acquiring contentment with his limited capacity, but school had begun to find him out. His body's increase in height and muscle bulk were now demanding more oxygen. The promise of the Glenn shunt was that it would produce better oxygen levels at rest, hence less blue colour, more pink, and hopefully better exercise tolerance. The main barrier was the massive procedure needed to get there.

Malachy came to the view that for quality of life, enough breath to walk uninterrupted between classes would be helpful. Class, after all was a theatre of entertainment. The young man who had struggled so much through his first decade of life was finally becoming well known for qualities other than breathlessness.

Niamh and Seamus both knew him as a fun companion, always willing to join in whatever game or joke was on offer. Niamh was now in Year 10, her first year of boarding school. She had passed both her mother and her older sister in height and was rising to the challenge of making new friends in the singular atmosphere of the convent boarding house. Her shy, reticent manner belied her great range of talents. I felt her to be unnecessarily modest, like both her older siblings. Niamh was a gentle soul, with a keen empathy for underdogs, perhaps born of growing up so close to one.

Seamus had always been remarkably popular with his peers and developed a wide cohort of good friends through high school, but remained an unruffled companion to Malachy, completely untiring in his willingness to share games with his brother. This entailed unyielding resistance to parental entreaty to spend his time more constructively. The boys needed limits set on their endless Teenage Mutant Ninja Turtle battles or games of Wii Soccer, as Seamus refused to allow the study demands of the HSC examinations to intrude on his Malachy-time. Study somehow could always wait until he returned to school.

Imogen also had a close bond with Malachy, whose mental wiring seemed to match hers in some ways. He proved the exception to her general reluctance to personal closeness. Since heading off to boarding school Imogen had rarely shown much emotion to either Maggie or me, and tended to steadfastly demonstrate her lack of neediness. That all came crashing down as 19-year-old Imogen, in her second year of university, cried on our shoulders in fear and anxiety for her brother approaching his operation. The strain pushed her to decide to take a short break from her studies that year.

Our family were not alone in feeling Malachy's charismatic appeal. The school yearbook for 2013, the year of Malachy's operation, includes some commentary from his classmates. Some of the comments bring home how people saw Mac's depth of character, and how complex and interesting he was:

'Malachy. He isn't an average kid. He is a very unique individual. He has a very interesting taste in clothing. He always knows how to make you happy, even when you think it's not possible.'

'He made me love life when I just couldn't. I remember when I got my headphone splitters and first brought them to school. Malachy LOVED the idea of sharing his music with me...'

'He will always love Harry Potter, a boy set apart from others since before he could remember for something he wasn't aware of ... his magic was being such a great and good person despite all of the challenges he faced.'

'Malachy [is like] a brother ... We ... fight about stupid things like government or ties and bow ties. He could always make everyone happy on a rainy day.'

'With Malachy, everybody is special, unique, loved and befriended. I didn't need to know Malachy long for us to connect and talk about life. No matter how hard his life, he would make mine better.'

'[Malachy is] talented, funny, smart and so much more.'

The tributes bring a smile, as the quirkiness we so loved in our domestic entertainer was clearly shining through in his school life. Among the anecdotes and profession of virtues was plenty of the cheeky stuff too, the stuff you don't want the teachers to know you're secretly proud of, the bits a parent with high expectations doesn't necessarily want to know:

'... your crazy antics and your intelligent mind ... your colourful ties.'

'Malachy ... a great friend to have in most of my classes. (makes) the classes fun and (telling) lots of jokes and stories ... saying "swag" in class.'

'[Malachy does] things at large, even down to the jokes... (He never told one that wasn't funny.) ... a free spirit who (thrives) on the laughter of others (often causing the laughter himself) and he never (stops) making us smile.'

That Malachy, the one who 'never stops making us smile', 'no matter how hard his life' was the version of Malachy to the fore that March day at Westmead hospital as the clock ticked down and the gas and needles hovered. Choosing to be high on the attention rather than levelled by fear, he embarked on recounting a performance of one of his favourite comedians, Michael McIntyre. He bantered away as the anaesthetist set to work, at first just chattering into space, but with time enthralling his audience. Malachy relayed the tale of an English tourist taking a taxi ride through Dublin. He buzzed along as the joke expanded, drawing in Maggie, the nurse, and the doctor, as the climax approached. The drama centred around the escape of a penguin from the Dublin zoo coinciding with a prison escape on the other side of town. The joke built and built and the professionals paused, suspending their work for the punchline to fall. A pregnant moment hung in the air as Mac drew breath for the final knockout blow:

'AND THE TAXI-DRIVER SAID—'

At that moment, to the dismay of his audience, Malachy succumbed to the sedation of the drugs.

Yet again, Maggie and I stared down our inner turmoil as we surrendered our child into the hands of the medical professionals. Again, there was the forced leap of faith, while we could do nothing for Malachy, we had to believe he was in the best possible hands for the interminable minutes or hours that would follow.

A truism it may be, but I felt determined to honour the belief of the stoic philosopher, Seneca, that nothing could be achieved by worrying. At another level I wanted to role-model coping with Malachy's Malady, because if Maggie and I, at the centre of the drama were inconsolable, what hope did others have of lending meaningful support?

Fear was the elephant in the dining room as we pensively chewed on our meal at the hospital cafeteria, trying not to picture Malachy's Glenn shunt procedure. He was on the operating table, chest stretched open straining his ribs, his blood on the sterile drapes and on the gloves of the surgeons, his lungs rising and falling with the hiss of the ventilator. Maggie and I had seen Imogen off, home to work on her difficult maths. We covered our anxiety with light, long forgotten conversation. Other diners seemed to be doing the same. Time moved slowly, expectation hovered in the air between us, for one, then two hours. At three hours the phone rang.

He'd made it through.

Pushing our plates aside, whatever topic we had settled on was washed away by a tsunami of relief. Springing from our chairs, Maggie and I hugged each other.

The operation is hard for parents, but for the child, who throughout surgery is anaesthetised into an oblivious dream world, it is the recovery that hurts most. Mac returned to intensive care a narcotised mess of tubes, drains, wires and bloodied dressings. A bank of drip stands delivered the poisons required to push his blood pressure up, to push his blood pressure down, to make his heart pump harder, to dull his pain, to help him sleep. Further connections to medical equipment caught the fluids that left his wounded chest, and fed back sterile fluid to hydrate his cells, and monitored his breathing, pulse, blood pressure, fluid output, oxygen levels, and heartbeat. We gazed on, relieved by the rise and fall of his chest. Its cadence signified life resumed, and what's more this time life was resumed with better plumbing than Malachy had ever known. There was still a hazardous path to recovery ahead for Mac.

The bedside days in intensive care passed slowly, the steady rhythms of Malachy's breath and heartbeat were interrupted intermittently by alarms and warnings, rounds of nursing observations or the march of the doctors' ward round. Occasionally the intensive care bubble was popped by visitors, all greatly relieved to see Malachy pulling through with only a routine amount of drama. As he roused into consciousness Malachy woke to the realisation that, painful as it might now feel, his operation had been successful. He was rightly proud that he'd had the courage to proceed, despite knowing the pain and risk involved.

Day one after waking produced a frightening moment as Malachy, stiffly trapped in place by his cables and tubes, unable to speak for the ventilating tube in place, stared maniacally at the empty space between Imogen and myself. Stretching one long domed finger as if to a ghost he pointed at … what? We looked behind us to find the source of the terror but saw nothing. This prompted further frantic gesticulation from Mac, clearly distressed by our incomprehension. With more animation we turned, clarified the absence of any being or object in the direction he was glaring. Everyone in the room hoped Mac hadn't developed hallucinations, which would be a tragic turn for a boy who'd suffered enough. I drifted closer hoping to reassure the terrified looking Mac of my unyielding love. He lunged at me, missing my arm by millimetres, I leant forward to clasp his hand in solidarity, he grabbed again, securing my left wrist in his grasp. He turned my wristwatch toward his eyes and nodded. The time: all he wanted was to be told the time!

Two days passed with us trapped within the singular logic of paediatric intensive care, in which you can eat all the ice you want but can only drink water in increments of ten mils per hour.

Deeming both ice and the liquid form to be equivalent quantities of water, I conspired with Mac to pass him more than the officially allowed liquid, with thirst being his constant companion. Ten millilitres may be a lot of liquid to a tiny newborn, but not to this patient. Seeing Malachy stretched out unconscious on the bed brought home one thing loud and clear. Our baby was now man-sized.

This fact brought with it additional challenges in the paediatric setting, where nursing staff are accustomed to the innocent hairless bodies of babes and infants, who have no coyness in the face of rudimentary nursing care. Once you add a deep broken voice and some pubic hair, the sensitivity of everyone increases. Three days into his recovery Malachy no longer had a urinary catheter, so it fell to him to voluntarily pass urine into a flask. Lying supine as he was, it proved beyond him to produce anything, despite the urge to go. Ultrasound was used to confirm a full bladder, and the pressing need for it to empty. Given his failure while lying down, this would now be the impetus to push Malachy to stand for the first time since his surgery. The task would involve ample pain, eased by the clutching of pillows and blankets to his healing sternal wound. It would need support and observation to make sure he didn't collapse from pain or low blood pressure or some other unforeseen complication. All of a sudden, the nursing staff disappeared, ordaining that as the only male person present, I was qualified to help my son urinate into the bottle. Of all the times for prudery to rear its head! Malachy stooped at the edge of the bed, clutching his chest, while also trying to steer the hoped-for stream of yellow fluid with a spare hand. His slight form curled forward as I gently held him across the shoulders. He strained and waited, and strained and waited.

No wee in an intensive care environment meant the certainty of needing placement of a urinary catheter. Suddenly no one felt qualified to help Mac empty his bladder, and the call went out for the only male nurse on the shift to rush to our aid. It would seem strange in the world of adult hospitals, but there it was; female paediatric nurses didn't do teenage catheters. As the only other available male, I was left to be the assistant to the procedure. The nurse, for his part, fumbled uncomfortably with the apparatus, clearly inexperienced, and perhaps nervous at being left to fly solo with the sensitive task. Being male doesn't automatically qualify someone to catheterise. In the end it was lucky I was skilled at urinary catheterisation as I was forced to take over from the poor bloke to complete the job. As amber fluid flowed the strain on Malachy's face faded.

For the rest of that week Malachy made steady progress, leaving behind his various tubes and supportive medications until he was no longer in need of such intensive nursing.

Relatively unencumbered, though still sore and fragile, Mac was freed to the fresh air and less monitored environs of the ward.

41

NO MIRACLE, BUT...

It is a waste of time to be angry about my disability. One has to get on with life and I haven't done badly. People won't have time for you if you are always angry or complaining.

— Stephen Hawking

S trange as it may seem, escaping intensive care for the freedom of the ward is not easy for families. While the doctors or the protocols have deemed your child no longer needs all the paraphernalia of life-saving machines, it is at first hard to feel sure of this. As they wheel your child from the ICU you forego having your own nurse, closely attentive to your child, and your child alone, all hours of the day and night, and the back-up of alarms to promptly draw attention to any imperfections. All that monitoring and scientific certainty is replaced by comparatively very little attention at all.

Malachy woke in the strange new surrounds of his own room on the Edgar Stephen Ward at Westmead. He was propped up at 45 degrees in bed as he turned to his left to look towards the courtyard. He groaned as his twisting movement wrenched one bony surface of his sternum against the other. The chest wall would take many weeks to stabilise. Feeling an irritation or a film of secretions move within his airway he coughed before his eyes widened in pain. I jumped to his side from the comfort of the bedside chair, where I had sat reading, waiting for the bustle of daily hospital life to begin. Malachy's every movement was slowed by the aches of surgical wounds, the constraint of oxygen tubing and the ever-present intravenous lines.

Thus started a long day that would later see Malachy instructed in the method of pressing towels to his chest before moving his body or clearing his throat. This was a day in which he would learn at the careful instruction of the physiotherapist the technique of huffing and prolonged expiration to clear his chest with the least possible blasting power. A day which would also see him make it through his first post-operative shower, while I hovered, fearing his frailty or that some flaw in the newly sewn plumbing of his heart may lead to a spell of fainting. Malachy agonised his way through the washing, then the towelling, and slumped into a plastic chair, exhausted yet refreshed in the perfumed aroma of cleanliness.

What this cost him in effort and strain was scarcely apparent as the day got moving, with a parade of professionals in and out of the room. Meals were delivered but mostly ignored for want of appetite. Medications were swallowed and observations made. A stream of doctors requested use of Malachy's body for their further training—to hear the sound of his heart murmurs, to impress their mentors with diagnostic skill in the history and examination. Not once did Malachy refuse a request to lend himself to the learning process. Not once did he complain, though I knew what effort it was taking just to shift in his bed or turn his head. He gladly accepted any pampering his parents would offer and was at times frustrated that we could not quite get those pillows right, but once the door swung open the outsiders only saw Mac the stoic. It was the same kind of generosity we would later hear he showed his friends, where despite nearing his own limits, he would sometimes carry a school bag for a limping classmate or help push a wheelchair.

Pink was the desired colour, and by the time he escaped the hospital toward the end of March, Malachy had nearly achieved the optimal hue. In heart healthy children the oxygen saturation reading is 98 to 100 percent. Malachy's levels, which had hovered down in the low seventies pre-operatively settled into a new range in the 80s. I had an uneasy feeling that after all the build-up to surgery, the deferral and the eventual plunge, Malachy seemed underwhelmed. In all the kerfuffle, I may have missed that what Malachy was after was complete normality—100 percent saturation. Normal exercise ability. Deep inside, I too, was hopeful of a more obvious transformation than what we saw.

Mac didn't have a truly dramatic renewal but there was still the consolation of a number of reasons to believe the new circulation was the best available. The new structure was right, but the unknown element was just how much efficiency Malachy's damaged heart and vessels could extract from the modification.

I feared for his emotional well-being as Malachy wrestled with the possibility that the years of planning and waiting, judging to perfection the minutiae of potential benefit, and weighing it against the risks had left him feeling something akin to Peggy Lee's: 'Is that all there is?'

Maggie and I watched for the signs that would tell us how he had fared. Was his life any better? Was he happier, more mobile, more energetic? We felt there was progress. Mac's vaunted resilience risked masking the downside. He was so stoic we didn't know whether he would complain if his outcome was poor. As our uncertainty dragged on past Malachy's eventual return to school, we spent long hours wondering, discussing and hoping.

Two weeks into the school term Maggie heard the front door swing open, and the shuffle of feet and bags as Malachy arrived home with his great mate PJ, an inspirational and dedicated friend, who on this day as most days had carried two school bags up the hill from the bus stop: his own and Malachy's. Malachy, still in a long process of rebuilding his strength seemed less worn by the short walk than usual.

'Hello, boys. How was your day?' Maggie enquired as they trudged down the hall.

'Fine. It was okay,' the boys understated in unison.

Then, 'Oh, yeah, Mum!' exclaimed Malachy. 'I made it to K Block without a break.'

Satisfaction grinned its way across the room as the meaning of this sank in. The failure to reach K Block had been the last straw that inspired Mac's choice to proceed to surgery. Now Malachy had made it.

This was a resounding symbolic victory. If it achieved nothing more, the operation had hit this poignant target. A Year 8 student, a youth of 14 years, could now walk to class.

Could he run with his friends and play the sports he so craved on his darker days? No, but years of struggle had taught him resilience, and he carried this quality like a trusted shield into the battles ahead. We would learn that the human qualities of this puny little guy were in demand in the schoolyard. Mac's absence had not been plain sailing for his friends, who were used to the drive, the humour and the unifying aura he brought to the group.

I met up with the parent of one friend who told me there'd been an incident. A bullying incident.

'It is such a shame,' she told me. 'If Malachy had been there, it wouldn't have happened.'

Her son, who had joined our conversation chimed in, 'I wish Malachy had been there. He wouldn't have let it get out of hand.'

Stunned and quizzical, I filed these thoughts away.

Days later the chance arose for me to ask Malachy about the incident.

'Mac, I heard there was a problem with the lads last term?'

'Yeah, Dad, there was a bit of an INCIDENT,' he intoned heavily. 'It's probably a bit of a misunderstanding, but they've been pretty upset. They had to have meetings with the principal, and the counsellor. Even the parents got involved.'

'Whoa, Mac, that's pretty bad. What's going on?'

'Yeah, it's bad, but you know, Dad, this might seem strange, but I know it wouldn't have happened if I'd been there.'

'What do you mean?'

'I don't know; I just know I could have kept them cool. It's hard to explain.'

Malachy, short of breath, unable to run and play but bearing some unknown magic. Magical charisma, a form of genius dedicated it would appear to the service of good, not evil!

Love him as they did, Mac's friends nonetheless were unable to carry his burden for him, and he'd grown enough in wisdom to see this, and sadly to reflect on the loneliness his affliction conferred. Only by living in his skin every day could anyone know what it meant for every gentle slope to seem a mountain, every game an endurance challenge, and every outing a feat of considered planning. Seamus, ever the receptacle of Malachy's thoughts, spoken or otherwise, was on hand for a reflective moment.

Malachy shared a hard-won insight.

'My friends are great. They care about me a lot, I know.'

He paused, briefly daunted by the intimacy of his reflection.

'My friends don't REALLY understand. They can still go off and do things I can't. They don't have to LIVE with it.'

His friends were not alone in that. I try not to cringe when I remember some of the debates we conducted around Mac's abilities and obligations. We walked a fine line between demanding normality of our distorted reality and resigning to defeat. It is the line we tried to manage of giving an 'abnormal' child a 'normal' life. Sometimes I got caught up trying to force unwanted normality on Mac.

Year 8 at St John the Evangelist is a time loaded with personal development goals. Students learn to look out for their friends, avoid drugs, pregnancies and sexually transmissible diseases, to value their loved ones and understand their inner strengths. Among the efforts to communicate these worthy values and life skills, St John's conducts an event called 'Empower Me Day'. It's a great day, tailored to the cultural challenges of teenagers. The activities on offer as Malachy approached his date with empowerment had a gendered flavour to them. To exaggerate for clarity's sake: Boys confront their fears and open up over a rock climb or an abseil, while girls form groups to analyse social pressures and how to manage their media-fuelled urges to anorexia and depression. Malachy was stuck, he was physically incapable of doing the 'boy stuff' while the 'girl stuff' had absolutely no relevance for him. Rightly or wrongly, he took the path of school refusal, immediately drawing advice from all sides of the dinner table.

Imogen and I sided with a sense of duty and obligation, suggesting he should front up regardless, that truancy showed a lack of civic sense. Against strident protest from Malachy, we suggested this was all part of the deal. You have to live with the heart disease, so you have to choose a suitable activity. Tension rose in the kitchen, as the importance of feeling locked out and misunderstood on account of his disability thrust itself to the front of Malachy's thinking. Maggie was softer on Mac, having her own doubts about the social stereotyping of the programme. Countless tiny incidents of soft treatment to accommodate Mac no doubt loitered in the background as Imogen, who had taken just three sick days in her 13 years of schooling, felt piqued by the unequal expectations. Maggie read the play a few steps ahead of the rest, seeing Malachy's growing aggravation she eased out of the fray, realising that our support on this issue meant a lot to Mac. Tears welled in her eyes as it dawned that Malachy was being asked to add yet another day as an outsider to the events of his peers. Mac blew his stack at Imogen and me.

I reason that inequities are unavoidable in a family so marked by profound disability. As much as Maggie and I tried to protect Mac and the others from the impact of his higher needs, we couldn't be perfect. Though it rarely blew up, there was strain on all sides.

There was no winner in that fight. In the end Mac did go to school, with an adjusted programme, 'Empowering up' over a drum lesson before watching the other boys enjoy their abseiling adventure.

42

FAMILY LEGEND

Truly I tell you, if you have faith as small as a mustard seed, you can say to this mountain, 'Move from here to there', and it will move. Nothing will be impossible for you.

— Jesus of Nazareth

Tucked away in the corner of my mind, hidden by protective layers of life as we know it, is a painful memory. In the early darkness of a winter night my 13-year-old-self steps away from the family car. The door thunks closed as I straighten myself and set myself for the walk into the hospital. Dad is on edge, as he has been for days. I can still feel the bitterness of the night, and nature's sense of loneliness, for the couple of eucalypts struggling to survive against the bitumen of the carpark. Huddled against the light breeze, our group made its way into the harsh neon of the hospital foyer, jarring with its clinical promise. The promise of first-world medical science. The promise of cure.

Dad, who often worked at Hornsby Hospital knew the way and led us with surety to the ward. A grey-haired matron, officiousness tempered by familiarity, advised of the visiting restrictions, while my father, distracted, made his way to the room.

'Only two at a time. No noise. You have FIVE MINUTES each, FIVE minutes.'

'Thank you, sister,' was the unanimous response.

Age having some privilege, I was in the first pair permitted to enter. My mother's black hair fanned out on the pillow with uncharacteristic decadence. Mum lay, still, on her back, unresponsive. I hugged her, as if force of will could convey my love and mysterious healing power in a way that words and medicine couldn't. The hospital smell, formalin and cleanliness, with a hint of human sickness filled the room. I sought in vain for a response from my mother, and felt an alarm ringing deep inside. This is the alarm I've left stowed in that corner of my mind all these years. Sometimes its noise echoes in the distance, hollow and spare, sometimes it comes to the fore. Too loud to ignore, too serious to dwell on. At the time I didn't know how to manage the worry this 'alarm' signified. So I ignored it.

As with many significant moments, the importance of this one was lost on me. Thankfully.

Suffering had played only the most minor of roles in my life to that point. Had I really understood, I don't know if 13-year-old me could have handled the enormity of my mother's viral encephalitis. Some of what Mum would lose in those days of coma would never return. A 40-year-old woman would lose all of her memories and most of her language. A husband and seven children would lose the wife and mother they had known.

After days spent mainly in inert unresponsiveness it was established that Mrs Frawley had a virus destroying parts of the temporal and parietal lobes of her brain. As viruses are unaffected by antibiotics, there was no known cure, but there was a new drug, not much tried in Australia, in a new class. The new drug was antiviral. Acyclovir was an unknown entity, hence perfect for Mum's situation with death more likely as the virus raged on. My father agreed to a trial of the unknown drug.

As Mum slumbered on with limited consciousness, word of her plight got around. Given her precarious state and the faith of the family, one of our favourite priests made his way to the bedside. Father King was a much-loved figure at my school. Impeded by the obvious kindness of his nature, he was notoriously incapable of controlling classrooms full of boys. He was known also for his special dedication to the sick, with stories abounding of his apparent potency in the faith-healing arts. Family legend records the wonderful moment when the much-loved priest entered the sterile confines of the comatose woman's hospital room. My mother, to this point unmoving, rolled to face the visitor, then sat up and fixed him with her dark brown eyes.

'Hello, Liz, it's Kevin King here.'

'Hello, Father, thank you so much for visiting.'

My mother received Holy Communion, with a priestly blessing, uttered the correct pleasantries, then resumed her coma. The 'Miracle' has been enshrined in family folklore, even making its way into print in my father's autobiographical work, *A Surgical Life*. An agent of Jesus, an ordained successor of the first apostles, had brought a miraculous cure into our life. As the trans-substantiated body of Jesus was brought into the room, an all-powerful God had intervened to wake the sleeping woman.

So the story goes.

Miracles were intermittently topical in the parenting of Malachy, with various people offering their opinions regarding what a miracle it was he'd come as far as he had. This was a commonly proposed view. Less common was the idea a miracle either had occurred to save him at some earlier point, or, rarer still, that one may be in store for his future. Clearly for Malachy, as for my mother, an interventionist god could have much to offer.

I was not naturally disposed to a belief in miracles, despite my Catholic faith. As a six-year-old I had been stunned by the revelation that, 'With enough faith, you can move mountains'. I heard this eternal truth from Matthew's Gospel at mass one Sunday in 1972. I soon had use for the power of faith. I made the fantastic discovery that little lizards could be held up by the tail and would dance frantically back and forward to escape. It was great fun, until my lizard snapped in half and fell to the ground, unmoving. I was devastated until I remembered the solution was at hand. Gathering the two lizard fragments together I placed them in my top drawer, carefully bound in layers of tissue. Retiring to bed I huddled in a ball and prayed. Prayed with certainty. Prayed with fervour. Prayed with absolute unwavering faith for God to restore the creature I had slain. I woke the next morning excited by the knowledge I'd held my end of the bargain.

The trail of ants winding up the chest of drawers I shared with my brothers told a different story. Then I did cry. Not just for the death of my reptilian playmate, but also, though I didn't yet know the word, I cried for the death of God's omnipotence. I had encountered what philosophers and theologians refer to as 'The Problem of Suffering'.

Despite not having the words to explain it, I had a distinct sense that day that God was not as powerful as people claimed. Thirty years later, the incident resonated when I read something by David Hume the eighteenth-century philosopher. Hume's argument ran something like this: God is said to be all powerful AND all loving. But the world is unfair, and full of needless suffering. So why doesn't God take action? A loving God with power would erase all suffering. If God loves humans, He must not have the power to help them. If He has the power, He must not have enough love to use it.

Hume's words from two centuries earlier seemed to distil my childhood dismay at God's impotence.

Whatever hopes I had for Malachy, my life had taught me not to look for a miracle.

So, what happened to Elizabeth, my Mum? She survived her ordeal, physically intact but a changed woman. Seven children still had their mother, an altered mother. Saved was the loving nature, resilience and humour, gone were the words, the memories, the initiative and the drive. Saved was the driver's licence, if not the road rules. Caring for and cooking for her children eventually recovered, if not the familiar recipes.

My father, loyal to a fault, was driven into isolation by the demise of the original version of his best friend and beloved companion. The people who rallied in support of our beleaguered family could not replace Mum's lost ability to find and engage the friends of the past, or recapture the expected life ahead, now evaporated. Mum had been the social one. The two-way street of intimate dialogue between Mum and Dad would be one way thereafter.

Mum's partial recovery always struck me as more likely the benefit of hurried access to acyclovir than a heavenly miracle. Omnipotence for me is the power to fix things, miraculously, rather than patch someone up to limp through into dotage.

'What if?' for Mum. 'What if?' for Mac. It is too dangerous to contemplate the difference a truly miraculous cure would have made to our extended family. If Liz and Malachy had been the recipient of miracles, they were decidedly half-baked miracles.

The headline act of miraculous divine intervention is not what any of our lives are built around. Scepticism about God's interventionist power didn't stop me from enjoying very enriching involvement with the Church. Our whole family has had wonderful care, nurture and sometimes profound inspiration from our involvement in the community of faith. Maggie and I are fortunate to count a number of priests and members of religious orders as friends. Among them some of the most life-affirming, generous, selfless and wise people anyone could wish to know. Their faith helps them do so much for other people, that I don't quibble about how powerful their god might be.

It is a paradox that Maggie and I have found valuable to manage with sensitivity. Many values we ardently believe in, and consider universal values, were passed on through the faith. Our senses of wonder and of justice were born and cultivated in the context of religious faith. Catholicism at its best is our spiritual home and our culture.

On the other hand, my mind is much better suited to radical scepticism, and our life experience has educated against the powers of an interventionist God. Once Bertrand Russell and Charles Darwin worked their way into my thoughts, I couldn't help ranking philosophy above inherited dogma. Hume and Descartes' church of reason tells me more about the world as it really is.

A clear sense of reality was what I found most helpful in facing up to challenging times, but the God of Good Outcomes would always have a place in my heart.

Malachy was embraced within the community of faith. His deep respect for several men of the cloth was a testament to their formative involvement in his life, and the models of service, poise and contentment that he saw in them. If faith could move aside the mountain of childhood heart disease, then all the better.

For better or worse Malachy's life, like everyone else's, had to be lived in this world. Not as we want it to be, not as we hope it will be, but as it is.

43

LIFE IS FUN

The purpose of life is to live it, to taste experience to the utmost, to reach out eagerly and without fear for newer and richer experience.

— Eleanor Roosevelt

Malachy's 'real world' operation didn't deliver the normality he dreamt of but there was a new vigour and purpose about the post-operative Malachy, now past his fourteenth birthday. It may have been simply that the burden of decision had been lifted; whether perfect or not, this was the new deal, the circulation that was designed to see him through into adult life. Malachy's circles of friends expanded as he broadened his hobbies.

He shared his new-found passion for drumming with a mate at school, while slowly working away at his skills at home. Drama added a new dimension, with weekly sessions at the Nowra Players providing the chance to share some creative space with a gathering of like-minded peers. Malachy was usually found in animated dialogue with two or three fellow players, often including his new mate, Thor. I became reluctant to arrive on time to collect him, half feeling I was interrupting the expansion of his networks.

In this period of accelerated understanding and willingness to taste what life offered, Malachy enjoyed a 'not exactly a date' night. While we acknowledged the gentle protest that it wasn't a date and they were just friends, Maggie and I agreed that Malachy took particular care preparing for a trip to the movies with Camille, his travelling companion on the 7:30 bus.

Odd at that time for a young man his age in Nowra, Malachy donned a collared, long-sleeved shirt above his skinny jeans. The jeans were standard. What other jeans could a bloke of his build wear? The collared shirt less so in a community of jeans and T-shirt lads. Even odder was the tie, still rarely seen on the local scene unless worn by one of Malachy's friends or possibly the occasional imitator. Windsor knotted and tied in place just so, with his cuffs tugged straight sitting just beyond the sleeve of his light jacket, Mac looked smooth. I pointed out for completeness' sake that he'd be the only dude in a tie at the Roxy.

'I know, Dad. That's what I'm wearing.'

All good then. 'Okay, mate. I'll drop you down there. Are you meeting at the cinema or somewhere else?'

'Just to the Roxy, D-Money.'

The movie they saw that night was one of the Iron Man franchise. Superficially, it was more mainstream than Malachy's usual taste, but the quirkier stuff tends not to get a long run at Nowra's Roxy, so it ticked enough boxes to be the chosen 'non-date' movie.

In a perfect world, Malachy may have preferred something with more appeal to his off-beat humour. We were growing accustomed to him sharing his joy at eccentrically styled cinema. He loved the outsider's view of directors like Wes Anderson, who created for example, *Moonrise Kingdom*, with its drama centred on two strong-willed eccentric outcast young scouts. Apart from the off-centre characterisation, Anderson's movie offered beautiful aesthetic layering, with much of the cinematography able to be frozen into self-contained works of visual art.

Malachy's infectious delight with things that struck a chord meant we were usually abreast of his latest discovery. Alongside *Moonrise Kingdom*, Malachy enthused about another post-modern antiheroic fable called *Submarine*. If Malachy's potential coming of age had its awkward points, it was nothing compared to those experienced by Oliver Tate, *Submarine*'s central character. It fascinated me that the Bildungsroman genre would so captivate Malachy who seemed to identify strongly with the rocky paths traversed by the central characters.

Malachy used film to capture some of the fits and starts of puberty and adolescence. He did some filming on a weekend when the rest of the family were out of town. The footage shows Malachy beaming at the camera, bursting with the excitement of friendship free of parental oversight. The hand-held camera is passed around the room, where there is a constant flurry of banter, riffing away with two of his friends. The boys are seen sharing the joy of new music, dancing to it, on the air guitar, heedlessly acting up for the camera. They are creating perfect embarrassing material the likes of which might resurface for speakers at subsequent milestone events. Malachy at one stage laughs so hard his face turns dark blue, and hiding his exhaustion, he flops to the ground, where his laughter can continue with less physical effort. The happiness of the boys is infectious. Malachy looks completely unafraid and blissful.

The soundtrack to the manic pleasure is Bloc Party's *Ratchet*. It is a song with a repeated crescendo of euphoric guitar noise, pushing the excitement from a low to a high simmer, and back. The ebb and flow of excitement mirrored my feelings as I watched the recording. On reflection, it was also mirroring that period in Malachy's life, when with his surgery completed, his euphoric sense of fun bubbled up and down incessantly.

Many days when I arrived home from work Malachy would be engaged in discovering some new act of genius from a young YouTuber or from a musician or band. Some days he would be buzzing to relay something a friend had said or done. At other times he'd be abuzz with some creation or thought of his own. Day upon day he seemed to be picking pearls out of the world's oysters.

After one weekend away Malachy described a party he'd attended with the family he'd stayed over with. Mac's friend was a fairly new friend he'd made through drama classes, and we didn't know his parents very well. They moved in different circles from us, heavily involved in the local arts crowd. Mac seemed adrift in his thoughts when we brought him at home on the Sunday night.

I greeted him: 'So, Mac, how was your weekend?'

'Good.' An atypically brief answer.

'Good?'

'Yeah, Mags and D-money, it was good.'

Such unaccustomed brevity invited a nudge from Maggie: 'Did you do anything interesting this weekend?'

'Nah, just hung out … Oh, wait, D-money, we went to the best party last night.'

'Mmm?' I turned to show my interest.

'Well, you guys would have loved it. It was all this arty crowd out in the bush. There was a fire juggler and old hippies and all these really cool people.' His head flicked slightly left then right, his eyes bright. He weighed his next description.

'There was this old hippy stoner guy. Picture him, Dad, with a long grey beard and a hippy vest, smoking a joint. He had some old-school tattoos and some piercings, looked like a Harley-riding old dude. It was straight out of the sixties. He was telling us how good weed is. How alcohol makes you violent but weed just mellows you out. It was like he was selling me a health food.'

This sounded outside our comfort zone. More than with any of our older children we dreaded Mac being drawn into drug use or other risk-taking behaviours. The risks were multiplied by his disease. Having sheltered him so carefully, I was concerned the old stoner may have frightened Mac. So I wanted to hear more. 'Sounds like a pretty interesting party, Mac.'

He went on, 'I was like, "Oh, yeah, tell me more". It was so great, Dad—I'm putting him straight into a story.'

There was no shock or fear. To Malachy the wayward characters were more human sketches to feed into his writing. He was a 14-year-old experience-sponge at work.

'That arty crowd sure are interesting, Dad. There were heaps of really nice people. The old stoner was the funniest though.'

Stoners, hippies, drunks and fire jugglers were all no problem. So I was fascinated to see how a different kind of threat, a movie night with a girl would work out.

I drove down the street to collect Malachy after the curtain fell on the Iron Man experience. Parking across the street from the cinema I scanned the dwindling crowd on the footpath. The bright lights of the Roxy's façade spilt onto clusters of teenagers, joking and chatting, saying their farewells. At the edge of the throng, I spotted my son. Standing typically straight, with a formality befitting his penchant for ties and collared shirts, he was fixed in animated discussion with his diminutive companion.

At my vantage point I paused, letting the moment sink in. This may not be the time or the person, but sure enough, my boy was old enough to fall in love. This boy for whom every milestone had once seemed unlikely had reached this point. The hormones of approaching adulthood were easing him forward, over that threshold into the life ahead.

Not wanting to spy, I climbed out of the car and crossed to greet the youngsters. We made small talk while waiting for Camille's mother to collect her. The two young friends seemed perfectly composed, relaxed in each other's company. Malachy didn't need me for anything but the ride home.

Without my realising it, they'd grown old. My precious son, whose every waking moment I had sweated on, was old enough to have secrets from me. He and his friend, were suddenly old enough to have their own shared understanding I wasn't party to.

Symbolic or real, in that moment I recognised that adult life was beginning. I could retire from helicopter parenting. With first the shaving, now a potential love interest, Malachy the Man had arrived.

44

SETTING SAIL FOR THE FUTURE

Most children feel immortal – they have no sense that they're ever going to die. For a child, even growing up is something that's barely comprehensible.

— John Saul

S eamus's final year of school was 2013. With life after school looming, every interaction he had with anyone other his immediate peers was tinged with expectation. Everybody's desire to know, 'What are you planning to do/hoping to get into, next year?' is a coded reference to the extent to which our culture is imbued with the idea that marks determine your success and direction for the rest of your life. The weight of having to know what career would make him happy forever, or fear that he couldn't work that out didn't visibly trouble Seamus.

The technique Seamus adopted to manage people's expectation was to avoid the question. He was content to reply, 'I don't know', but like any other academically inclined young person, he must have been wrestling to make a choice.

As the last holidays of his school career approached, he finally confessed to an ambition. Seamus wanted to study medicine. A brother living with a serious congenital heart defect proved to be quite an inspiration. Further questioning from Maggie elicited a suggestion from Seamus that he may in particular be thinking of becoming a paediatric cardiologist.

Whatever questions he'd never asked about his brother's illness, and the means of treating it, or the possible cures of the future, had been in his mind, they had never been voiced.

The holidays rolled around, to be followed by the all-important Trial examinations, which would form a large part of Seamus's ultimate mark. Medical degrees don't come easy; they demand entry marks galore. Naturally, we assumed a freshly inspired student would study like a man possessed through the final weeks of preparation. What we witnessed instead were more countless hours whiled away either playing with Malachy in Malachy's room, or doing the same in Seamus's room, with breaks to play Wii Soccer in the lounge room, with Malachy.

They didn't require any justification for the sharing of endless hours. Notwithstanding occasional skirmishes of brotherly hatred, accompanied by low-level violence, the friendship of the two boys was seamless. Malachy's gleeful lack of self-consciousness beamed from his face whenever Seamus returned home from boarding school.

I felt bothered that Malachy had trumped study in that last holiday period, knowing that Seamus would return to his exams under-prepared. I feel differently now. Overtaken by events and time, I place the greatest value on those intense periods of togetherness.

Trumping other concerns was one of Malachy's gifts.

The young man, Malachy, had emerged from the initial cauldron of years spent merely surviving his medical travails, then his later childhood adapting to the limitations of a feeble body and cupping the vicissitudes of a world built for the more able. Malachy, the man, was proving to bear almost no resentment towards his ill fortune. An infectious sense of delight walked with him. The qualities and challenges faced by others were every bit as interesting and as concerning to Malachy as his own.

I don't know what he looked for in people, what attracted him to some and not others, but it was clear he was heedless of the typical human prejudices. Your age or gender, your popular appeal or superficial attractiveness were not Malachy's yardstick. He reminded me of a description I recalled from my student days, when I read the acclaimed *Zen and the Art of Motorcycle Maintenance*. There is a passage intended to convey the sense of perspective often attributed to Indigenous people, whom you will hear (rightly or wrongly) have a tendency to divine the essence of a person. Credentials count as nothing in this framework.

The author of *Zen* is walking along a track with a Native American elder, a man of few words and reputed wisdom. A dog runs onto the path ahead of them, prompting the narrator to search his memory for canine breeds and the associated nomenclature. His upbringing and inclination can't be denied. He needs to ask, 'What type of dog is that?' The elder's reply is limited to the important information, 'It's a good dog'.

Interpreting people was something of an art form to Malachy, whom you could think of as a naive critic. If you tried to pin down his way of judging, it had shades of the style of wisdom of first nations people: 'I am no socialite, but I know what I like.'

At school people had grown accustomed to Malachy's free-ranging approach to social life. Many mornings he would drop by to hang out briefly with the school captain four years his senior. That young man is one person who has described feeling towards Malachy as if he were a brother.

In the lunch break he often spent some of his time with the Year 10 girls—Niamh's group of friends. Niamh was at boarding school in Sydney by this time, so there was a bit of a sibling demarcation war to be had. Niamh didn't want her little brother muscling in on her friends, 'little brother' being a recognised code for annoying hanger-on. Her friends on the other hand were entertained by Malachy and he in turn enjoyed their company.

Disabled children tug at the heartstrings, and to a young teenage woman the urge to care for someone can be strong, so it was no surprise Malachy quickly endeared himself to the older girls he encountered through his involvement in some of the school's drama activity. But he was past the age of, 'Ooh, he's so cute', and by temperament wasn't someone to be coddled. So as much as the older girls may have warmed to him with the aid of maternal instinct, dealing with Malachy forced you to deal on his terms. He wasn't fussed about crossing the barriers of age or gender. If he liked someone, he treated them as a friend.

I attended one of the school productions with Malachy in July 2013. As we bustled through the crowd to take our seats Malachy stopped to chat to a much older boy, one of the Year 12 students. The boy had the young surfer look, overgrown hair bordering on dreadlocks, well-tanned. I'd never met him. The matey repartee between them suggested they were quite familiar. Curious as to how Malachy knew the lad, I enquired. It turned out he was the boyfriend of a girl, three years Malachy's senior, who'd once been in his drama team.

Malachy somehow projected to people, 'I like you. You're cool and interesting.' People seemed to respond well and met him halfway.

I wasn't immune to his charms. He did something most teenagers avoid with intent. He made his father feel loved.

45

THE HUM OF DAILY LIFE

Perhaps we become aware of our age only at exceptional moments and most of the time we are ageless.

— Milan Kundera, *Immortality*

In 2013 Malachy was in Year 8 at St John's. His typical weekday included a bus trip to and from school, with his mate PJ acting as porter on the return journey. Arrival home would involve a bit of afternoon tea, then a turn at the computer with his friend. The computer would often be used for a war game of some description, with the two either teamed up or opposed, or used for admiring the genius of one or other young YouTuber or blogger.

In the evening, Malachy would share his day's discoveries with Maggie and me, and almost always report something interesting from school. He liked to discuss solutions to a problem at school, or a quandary in respect of his circle of friends. Invariably his concerns and preoccupations were to do with the welfare of someone other than himself.

Sometimes he returned to his thoughts about the fair distribution of talents within the group, implying a God who cared for his creatures would spread things a bit more evenly. Injustice was to be railed against, whether it occurred at the hands of human agents or at the unyielding hand of fate.

For a period, he worked on finding a way to bring someone back into the fold after they'd been marginalised in some way.

242

No one would be ostracised. Mac anguished over preserving harmony amongst his friends, finding ways to help the others to see that a minor personality flaw in anyone in the group, did nothing diminish the deeper character of the person.

Malachy would hate this story getting out, but it greatly affected both Maggie and me.

Reflecting on some of his best friends one day Malachy exclaimed, 'It's good that I have heart disease'.

Maggie was jolted to attention. We were not accustomed to associating the word 'good' with Malachy's dramatic course through life.

'Well,' his head tilted into thoughtful posture, 'you know how the others are good athletes? If I had a good heart, I think I would have been pretty good at athletics, maybe even better than my friends. But I'm not, so everyone has a chance to be the best. Some of my friends aren't so good at schoolwork and some don't make friends as easily as me, so it wouldn't really be fair if I was great at sport as well. This way everyone gets a turn to shine.'

Malachy was so unguarded and such a universal carer. His utilitarian streak made him an enemy of prejudice. Once, it had been his grave neonatal plight that moved us, then the numerous sufferings of his infancy. Now what moved Maggie and I was his personality.

Occasionally, Mac would return to the theme of his love of Vietnam, especially when our friend Hai, our tour guide in Vietnam, let us know he planned to visit Australia. Hai had sought approval from the communist regime to travel to Australia for a travel expo to promote his fledgling company, Absolute Vietnam Travel. We invited him to be our guest in Nowra, and to enjoy the Shoalhaven region as a tourist when he had the chance.

Once Hai arrived in Nowra, Malachy was stoked by Hai's assertion that he would cook some traditional food for us. Hai spent half a day finding the necessary stock and equipment and got down to the business of preparing what Malachy saw as his own slice of heaven on earth, a chicken pho. I took a photo of Malachy eating his pho, but such was his alacrity in consuming the delicacy I couldn't capture his face. The enthusiastic stoop of his head, as close as possible to the object of his desire, obscures his face. His chopsticks jut out, shovelling the noodle combination to his mouth. Mac's fingers gracefully curl in support of the sticks, tapering to the delicate blue domes, so instantly recognisable. His expression of delight at the meal was so obvious that Hai was left in no doubt how much Malachy appreciated his effort.

When our old car started to fail that year, we felt Malachy, with his strong tastes, had earned the right to help us choose a new one. For our trip to the dealer Malachy donned his skinny jeans, mismatching socks, bright coloured shoes, a collared shirt, and his much-loved Tweety Bird tie. When he went to deal, he went dressed to impress.

Comfortably dressed, Maggie and I wandered the car yard outclassed by our sharp-dressed offspring. We bumped into a friend from my cricket team there with his wife. Meeting Malachy for the first time, my friend was suitably impressed by the sartorial splendour on display. He made a point of engaging Malachy in conversation. The 14-year-old caught the man in conversation with his entertaining account of the sort of vehicle he was looking for. The main features Mac needed were space and comfort in the back row, where he would inevitably be forced to sit, and more importantly a decent sound system, with speakers near his seat. With his guidance, and half an eye on family road trip to Tasmania we chose a Kia Carnival.

Around that time Malachy had a routine check-up with Dr Cooper. The ultrasound of his heart looked much as expected, with just slight turbulence where the shunted blood returned to the heart but a good recovery from the operation. To my eye the main ventricle looked the same as ever, and this was confirmed by Dr Cooper's measurements. Mac mentioned an occasional flutter of palpitation in his chest, something he'd felt on and off for years.

It was no cause for alarm. He also described feelings of pressure in his chest, which is the type of description people give when they have heart-related pain. Maggie, Mac and I discussed it with Dr Cooper, who reminded us what we knew of Mac's anatomy. He had always had some difficulty getting enough oxygen to his heart, but had always coped. Dr Cooper pointed out that it's normal for Heart Kids to regulate their activity to deal with such symptoms. Mac was no different. If he felt heavy, he would ease off from any activity. The conclusion was that it might well be heart pain, but Mac had it in hand.

In the August, Niamh was at home and had organised to meet up with some of her old local friends at a cafe. Malachy invited himself to join in on the outing. The two of them set off down the street and had a great afternoon, sharing the company of the girls. Niamh later commented on how much fun it was, and how lucky she was to have an appropriately cool little brother. Malachy, too, felt lucky to have such closeness to a loving older sister with interesting friends who 'got' him.

The following weekend was the date of the annual HeartKids Tiny Tickers Ball which Maggie and I were attending in Sydney. Malachy wasn't yet old enough to be left to himself for the weekend but was fortunate to have Imogen taking a break from university that semester, and at home for the weekend. Imogen's closest friend was coming down for a visit. Imogen and Malachy had always shared a sense of humour and other kindred patterns of thought, but the bond between them had grown even more affectionate since the tension of Malachy's big operation earlier in the year. Mo, as we know her at home, is a great one for outings, liking to be busy and to extract the flavour from life.

Mo hatched a plan to head out to the bayside hub of Huskisson with her friend and Mac for a picnic. With the food spread on the grass in front of them and slanting sunlight illuminating their left sides, brother and sister posed for a photograph. Mo, sullen with mock seriousness has her left hand poised in a double entendre of

245

thumb raised, middle finger extended. 'All Good' meets 'The Bird'. Malachy, delighted with the day, the picnic, the company, mirrors her left hand with his right, but can't match the sombre facial expression. He beams happiness, unable to disguise his enthusiasm, even for artistic effect. Imogen and Malachy's heads lean in to meet as their sunlit middle fingers point each to the other. The image captures, beautifully, the kindred quirky natures of our eldest and youngest children.

46

IN THE BUS QUEUE

Adolescence represents an inner emotional upheaval, a struggle between the eternal human wish to cling to the past and the equally powerful wish to get on with the future.

— Louise J Caplan

September 3rd, 2013, was busy, like most days in our household Maggie was away that day. Work had sent her on a brief retreat, for staff development. She had spent two days reflecting with a group about many things, including her life as a mother to a seriously ill child. Imogen was home, taking a break from uni, but sleeping in that morning. So, I was in sole parent mode with Malachy. Mac had his usual rushed breakfast, and probably didn't have his daily dose of aspirin, a blood thinning ritual I was not always successful at enforcing.

Mac had either overslept, or intentionally eschewed his usual bus ride to school. The bus ride found him most days enjoying the company of two of his closest friends—his great neighbourhood mate PJ, and his ally and confidante, the gorgeous Camille. I drove him the ten minutes to school. I recall his slightly dishevelled bed hair, and his face in oblique profile as he walked away from me with a brisk affectionate, 'Laters, Dad', not knowing it would be the last time I would see Malachy conscious.

It wasn't like him to request a lift to school. Something about the bus weighed on him that morning. At one point in the morning

247

Malachy mentioned to one of his friends that he felt he needed to talk because he had a problem to solve.

In the lunch break he played basketball, which was not normal for Mac. Basketball was beyond his usual capability. Normally, Mac's approach to the game would be to rest until the ball came to him, then make a pass or shot before resting again. One friend told me, 'I had never seen Malachy run so far as he did in that game'.

After lunch Malachy felt sick, there was some of the familiar heaviness on his chest, but it didn't fade with rest in the usual way. One of his best friends discussed going to sick bay with Malachy, who on this day declined, instead persevering. He had spent many days in sick bay and didn't like to cause trouble.

What if Malachy had gone to the sick bay? What if?

He didn't look well in his afternoon class, but not looking well was something of a staple for Mac. Not long previously he'd been told by an unwitting teacher, 'You look like you've crossed over'.

His pale blue rejoinder that no, he merely had heart disease, must have produced a skipped beat or two as his identity dawned on the man.

Accustomed as he was to struggling on with symptoms, a heaviness here, a fluttering there, even a funny rhythm at times or transient light-headedness, Malachy pushed himself along, happy face to the fore, his oblivious thirst for life seeing him join the line for the bus. His earphones were in place as he selected the playlist of tunes for the trip home. His favourite tunes of the moment still included Bloc Party's *Ratchet*, and a handful by the Canadian indie producer Grimes.

With the escalating motif and accelerating tempo of *Ratchet* pumped into his ears, Mac turned to exclaim to his friend, 'Gee, I love this song'. Mac briefly clutched his chest as his body collapsed to the ground, his head striking the shoe of his friend. A music lover all his life, the five words 'Gee, I love this song' were the last he ever spoke.

Back at work I had grown accustomed to calls from St John's school put through by my secretary. Inconvenient but necessary, another discussion about poor old Mac, another decision to be made about whether to persist in class, wait for me at sick bay or consider other options.

This call started out much the same as others, 'Dom, it's Pieta. It's about Malachy'.

'Okay. What's he up to?'

'He's had a collapse at the bus line.'

'Okay, is he with you now? Do you want me to come and pick him up?'

'No.' Pieta paused, making a choking sound. 'Dom, he's had a collapse and they're still working on him. Bill is there and ... doing CPR... (I lost the words as shock overtook me) ...'

As we spoke, the school's head P.E. teacher was directing the attempt to resuscitate fallen Malachy. Other students were being ushered here and there, horrified by the scene unfolding.

There is a painful 'What If' right then. What I didn't say to Pieta that I might have said, were these words that haunt me by their absence: 'Have you got an automated defibrillator?'

I dropped everything, and ran to my car. My chest heaved with stress as I was trapped in the afternoon traffic of the Princes Highway. If road rage could part the traffic, I'd have shot through in record time. As it was, I inched my way there arriving just after the paramedics. Malachy was pale and ghostly still, as first the teaching staff, then the ambulance officers repeatedly compressed his chest wall to pump life-saving blood to his brain and kidneys. Shocked and remote, as in a dream, I thought all that could be done was being done and held back, letting the experts run their resuscitation. I was powerless to help or protect my child. I willed and hoped my presence would not distract the rescuers.

After 15 or 20 long, terrifying minutes I sat in the front passenger seat of the ambulance, my heart racing, my chest tight, while outside I was calm and rational. From the frantic interior of the rear cabin, where Malachy was being resuscitated, I heard the words, 'We have a rhythm'.

'GOOD ON YOU, MALACHY!' I yelled. Then, 'KEEP BREATHING, MAC. DEEP BREATHS, MAC.'

The paramedics said little as they stayed engrossed in a battle between life and death. Malachy had spent a long time without a native heartbeat, blood only circulating through the heroics of the prolonged cardiopulmonary resuscitation. I know this is bad, but hope is powerful. More so when it is all you have.

'KEEP BREATHING, MATE, KEEP BREATHING,' I yelled past the silence of the driver.

By the time our ambulance pulled up at the hospital it must have been close to an hour since Malachy expressed his joy at the sound of fresh music.

The typical result of such prolonged resuscitation is not impressive.

If I recall every second of that day, or that day and the one before, if I recall all the moments, all the little 'What Ifs' of my day, and all those I've now been told about, and then I go through them one by one, looking for something I can change, two things happen.

First, I find so many details I wish were different, so many tiny circumstances now burnt into my being that were ever so slightly wrong, ever so slightly different, that were invisible to me then.

Second, I find there is nothing I can change.

MALACHY'S MAGNUM OPUS

Esteban Devereaux's Adventure

Chapter Two (continued)
— Malachy Frawley 2013

2

Esteban sat down on a brick wall behind him and got his pants wet on the bricks that he hadn't realised were soaked in rain. **Oh. crap**, he thought, **I can't get up, now she'll think I'm weird.**

'You are weird,' she said

'What?'

'You talk to yourself; I heard everything you just said.'

'Oh.' He laughed at himself.

Several minutes later they reached the top of the hill and looked down into the wheatfields below. There was a large burnt patch and a faint glowing white light in the middle of it. Esteban could just make out a figure sitting cross-legged in the middle of the light. He and Lyris started heading down into the wheatfields. Going downhill was much easier for Esteban and they soon made it to the figure. Probably because Esteban slipped over halfway down, shortening his walking time dramatically. The figure sitting there was dressed in all white clothes. It was a he and he was very masculine and had a head of long curly blonde hair that was definitely too long for society's male hair-length expectations, but probably the strangest feature about him was that he sprouted beautiful, broad white wings that were as clean as Lyris' pants and although they were folded in nicely, Esteban estimated that they had a **pretty** big wingspan.

'Hello Lyris and Master Esteban,' he said in a deep and reverent voice. 'I bet you weren't expecting a visit from me,' he winked.

'No, not really, Gabe,' said Lyris.

'Wait you know this guy?' asked Esteban, 'Cos I'm still freaking out about the fact that he has wings.'

'That's probably expected,' said Gabe. 'Allow me to introduce myself; My name is Gabriel, the lord's messenger.'

'Are you an angel?' asked Esteban.

'Yes.'

'Okay, I'm officially freaking out now.'

'Would it help if I said, do not be afraid?'

'Probably not. So how do you know him, Lyris?'

'Oh, we go way back,' she said.

'I'm starting to get the impression that a lot should probably be being explained right now.'

'And, you'd be right. Why don't you sit down.'

'Speaking of which,' said Gabriel, 'Could you two please help me up? My landing was a bit rough.'

Esteban and Lyris helped Gabriel to his feet and saw that his ankle was twisted in an extremely bad direction.

'Why can't you just sprinkle some fairy dust on that and heal it?' asked Esteban.

'Don't be stupid,' said Gabriel, 'I can't use magic on Earth, any fool knows that.'

'Well, clearly I'm not just any fool,' Esteban retorted. He paused. The wheat behind him rustled and he could hear footsteps approaching. He turned to see a pack of teenagers about the age of seventeen arrogantly striding towards them, with the biggest, stupidest, cocky grins on their faces.

'Well, well, well,' said the quiff-bearing leader, slowly. 'Hello, Lyris, you're looking beautiful as ever.'

'Get lost, you ugly Satanist,' she said, 'or I'll skewer you.' She whipped a pair of wickedly sharp, diamond-shaped blades from the inside of her blazer.

'Whoa,' said Esteban. 'Those look dangerous, and, you know that guy as well?'

'Get behind me, now, Esteban,' she hissed.

'Right, your highness,' he said as he eagerly leapt behind her and stood next to Gabriel.

'Hand over the angel,' said the boy, his cocky grin fading and being replaced with a venomous glare and bearing teeth.

'Esteban,' Lyris said, 'take Gabe and get out of here while I take care of these guys.' She turned to the gang of boys and yelled, 'Come at me, bros!'

As she leapt towards them, slashing with her razor-sharp blades, slitting the throat of the first boy to charge at her, his blood splattered on the ground and stained the wheat and, in that instance, Esteban knew nothing would be the same for him again. This was not a dream, the cold air bit at him and the sun warmed his face; he was not sleeping, that he could be sure of.

He hefted Gabriel over his shoulder—the angel was surprisingly light considering his impressive build—and they started making their way through the wheat towards a large patch of trees that Esteban hoped they could hide in. After some time walking, someone cried out from right behind Esteban, and stupidly, he turned around to see one of the pack members fall to the ground, one of Lyris's blades sticking out of his back. Lyris was about to retrieve the blade when a pair of strong hands came from behind her and wrapped tightly round her neck. Lyris pulled at his hands but his grip would not loosen.

Esteban saw fright in her beautiful blue eyes and acted. He pulled the knife out of the boy on the grounds back and slashed at the hands around Lyris' neck. The boy cried out in pain and his hands withdrew. Lyris gracefully backflipped over him and twisted his head, snapping his neck, and instantly killing him. Esteban handed Lyris her knife as she yelled for him to 'keep going'. Esteban obeyed, fear pushing him onwards, but although he resisted it he could feel the need for a rest coming upon him. **No**, he thought, **not now**, but alas, he had to rest, so he sat down and watched Lyris fighting the last gang members.

God, she could fight. She flipped and kicked and stabbed, dropping low and ducking swipes from the ringleader, but as she ducked the ringleader raised his knee up hard and fast and it cracked against her chin, sending her sprawling. She lay there as the boy raised his sword, and he was about to bring it down on her. Esteban could not bear to watch, but at that moment Lyris looked up, and she had a ravenous, terrifying look in her eyes. The ringleader sprouted an incredibly unholy word as Lyris grabbed his sword with her bare hands and snapped it in two. Esteban could tell that whatever state Lyris was in now she was not human, she was something else entirely, something terrifying. Esteban just looked at her and was overcome with fright, he just wanted to curl into a ball and cower, but he didn't, he ran. Lyris pounced on the boys and tore them apart; blood and body parts flew everywhere, and although Esteban resisted it he vomited all over his sickly green clothes.

'Right,' said Gabriel, 'time to get the underworld out of here.' But it was too late.

Lyris charged towards them, there was no time to run, no time to do anything, Lyris pounced on Esteban and everything went black...

PART 4

DEMISE

Return to dust

47

BY MALACHY'S SIDE

Success is not measured by what you accomplish, but by the opposition you have encountered, and the courage with which you have maintained the struggle against overwhelming odds.

— Orison Swett Marden

To see my child asleep, breathing quietly, free of care, was a joy I anticipated long before having children to call my own. As a young man I had felt a strong sense of consonance with a John Irving character who would creep into the room of his dreaming children and simply feel the love.

When our first child was born, I felt so overwhelmed I temporarily lost regard for, or even awareness of myself. As if it were yesterday, I remember our daughter's first night in the world, when I had stayed at the bedside until she next woke, well into the next morning. Once that night Mo had flinched, her fingers sprung open, extended as if in surprise, then curled her fingers back to a neutral position, still but for the cadence of her breath, for five more hours. Cocooned in swaddling, one delicate hand peeping above the blanket, rosy lips unmoving she slept on in peaceful repose.

Almost 20 years later I found myself at the bedside of my fourth child, lying every bit as still, and serene. His arm stretched out the length of a man, not with the delicacy of a baby. I kept vigil on Malachy's fine features, moulded by his kind temperament, and his ever-growing love of people and their ideas. My love for Malachy is different from baby love, which is more of a hazy universal love for an unknown entity. Love for Mac was love born of deep knowledge. I watched this young man grow for fourteen and a half years, to now observe him lying serene, in the stillness of coma. As a family we had all ridden highs and lows with Mac, admired and enjoyed him, argued and played, and now we came to his bedside just to wait, and to be.

There are no furrows on his brow, no lines of worry, his sleep is deep, there is no sign of consciousness.

All I can offer my son is love, which now feels purposeful, as if I can will a change in the material course of what lies ahead. Again, I hardly feel my body, I care little for time, for food. I have no needs which can rise to the importance of Malachy's: to heal, to wake, to live.

Mac's face is beautiful at rest, his eyelids closed, with scurrying bouts of rapid eye movement suggesting there are dreams. I hope these dreams are sweet, that my child knows nothing of his predicament. As the hours pass there are comings and goings at the bedside because I am not the only one who loves this patient. As a family we keep this vigil together. As I hold Malachy, rest a hand on his chest, place his hand in mine, brush a wisp of hair back from his forehead, there is just one blemish, one clue to what has gone before: a tiny abrasion on his right upper eyelid belies the point of impact.

Malachy is not sleeping, he is in a coma, after his head struck the ground at the feet of his friends, marking him ever so slightly. Such a small 'tell'. How quietly disaster crept up on our child, unannounced and unexpected. As he rests, to the loving eye, the wound is near undetectable.

Malachy lies undisturbed, his coma assisted by medication, and by cooling his body. He is surrounded by his family: Maggie, Dom, Imogen, Seamus and Niamh. Any other purpose in life has become secondary to being present to our son and brother. Each life now changed forever regardless of the outcome. Along the way practicalities have needed tending—family and friends have been made aware of Mac's predicament. His reach is wide, and the urge for people to connect with his challenge is strong. Faces come and go at the bed and in the waiting areas. There are tears, hugs and phone calls. A myriad of people stepped forward each in their own way. Our gratitude is forever.

There seems no purpose in describing the medical road to this point. This was a time of pain, of trauma, the agony of fear, terror of the desperate consequences hanging over us. This was a time of prolonged resuscitation, ambulance rides, watching Malachy's body fail at each critical point—the CPR, the cardioverting 'shocks', the lines bearing fluid and drugs, blood samples, ventilating machinery, hours spent preparing for helicopter retrieval, then flying from Nowra to Westmead.

In these hours we each were hit by that wave of recognition; we each had the news reach us by one method or another. I had received that fateful call at work. Maggie and Imogen had been at home, with teachers from the school arriving at the door. Niamh was brought to the office of the boarding mistress to receive her news in company. Seamus similarly was at school, dragged from his planned birthday celebration to be told, 'Your brother collapsed at school; he is in hospital'.

48

A WEEK OF INTENSIVE CARE

Do not go gentle into that good night,
Old age should burn and rave at close of day;
Rage, rage against the dying of the light.

— Dylan Thomas

Six days in September 2013 took me through an experience of secret hope, flurries of expectation, bursts of sadness and joy, despair beyond desperation, and phases of frustration, exhaustion, gratitude and exasperation. For three days hope dominated. For one day it was uncertainty. For two days fortitude was all that was left.

For the first three days it was battle stations, everything that could be done was being done. Every medical support to ensure continued life was employed. Every test to gauge the success of this venture was performed. Every graph, image, and sound were scrutinised for evidence of return to 'business as usual'. The sweet relief of seeing life asserting itself once more was just around the corner of each new investigation. Kidneys working, tick. Heart pumping, tick. Lungs ventilating, tick. Brain responding to voice, maybe.

We had all stepped into another world. A tragic world of around-the-clock suffering. The ambient sounds of paediatric intensive care include the black-humoured banter of the nursing staff, arming themselves repeatedly against the weight of human tragedy that surrounds them. There is the hushed twitter of family conference, as doctors relay the latest judgment to expectant

259

hopeful families, desperate parents and carers, anxious siblings. The roll of trollies on the hard linoleum flooring echoes in the barren spaces within each room and disappears down the brightly fluorescent-lit corridors.

The unpredictable burst of alarms from monitors and pumps intermingles with the droll predictability of respirators, steadily sucking in and out with the rise and fall in the chests of the lying children. Muted greetings float through the halls as people balance duly sombre reflection on their dire predicament against the pleasure of reunion.

The sounds, the colours and the feel of that environment never leave you. The most horrible of realities are confronted there, beside the greatest saves, the steepest recoveries and the tide of relief they bring. The extremes of sadness in grief, and the ecstasy of escape or near miss are integral to the environment of intensive care. Even in my loss, the joy of earlier reprieves in that very same intensive care is readily summoned, complicating my bitter hatred of those days, my raging impotence in the face of the march of approaching death.

In this environment we waited, gradually meeting each of the doctors and nurses who would help Malachy along the way, seeking the information that might help us guess what lay just around the corner. The information we sought was the rays of hope, the possibilities of recovery, the signs of life resumed.

All the while Malachy lay suspended, his metabolism slowed by the intentional cooling of his body, his movement prohibited by the chemical straitjacket of muscle relaxants, all response subdued by sedative, combined with brain injury of unknown extent. All the while his heartbeat on, with no sign of whatever had happened to send it blank for that fateful hour. The organ which shaped and defined the challenges of this life of fourteen and a half years was acting, 'Nothing to see here, move along'.

While the heart beats, there is hope.

The heart, which got us into this mess, was no longer the vital organ. Nor was it the kidneys, which were filtering as new, the blood tests confirmed, nor the lungs, which with the help of extra oxygen were performing well enough to saturate the blood with the breath of life.

Vital to us now was the brain, so valued by Malachy as the source of his imagination, the source of drive and meaning when the body so often failed him. If the brain has died, the child is dead.

A technician arrived to perform an EEG (electroencephalogram). This is a test to look at brainwaves, the electrical activity of the brain. As Malachy lay there unflinching, comatose, patches of his scalp were gently abraded as the leads were pasted to his skull and the device began its graphic dance across the screen. Waves were there before our eyes. Does this mean life? Apparently not. Look for waves of response. What happens when we pinch his finger, or whisper in his ear? Does he respond to pain, to voice, to anything? Something changed when I spoke, my heart leapt as it seemed to be a response. I spoke again, and again the wave altered. Was he hearing me? That would need analysis by the doctors, but now I had something to sustain my hope. Some part of medical science was telling me, yes, he may have something ticking in there.

This information would need to be placed alongside imaging information, i.e. can we see normal brain tissue? Is there enough good brain tissue to mount a recovery?

For one day all that mattered was the answer to a simple question: does an MRI scan show Malachy's brain is okay? All else was put aside while Malachy was transferred downstairs for the scan, which if positive, would be the crowning success of all the work of resuscitation. Each of our lives now focused to this point, as we suspended all other considerations in favour of this moment of truth. Malachy's brain, I hoped, after a lifetime of low oxygen supply, might withstand the shock of an arrest better than normal.

Good news is often given publicly, at the bedside. Bad news is a private affair.

The scan was done, and the wait began. Eventually the message came through. 'We need to meet with the family.'

49

FROM CURE TO COMFORT

To be mortal is the most basic human experience and yet man has never been able to accept it, grasp it, and behave accordingly. Man doesn't know how to be mortal.

— Milan Kundera

What is there to say about interview rooms? Interviews are what made Michael Parkinson a household name, or made you feel you knew the star of an upcoming movie, or brought you insight into the creative mind of a guest on your favourite radio programme. Interviews also helped Scotland Yard know who to arrest, or helped you secure a job or choose a new employee. Somehow the word doesn't quite work for a meeting whose only purpose is for experts to tell desperately worried people what they don't want to hear.

Dread of the interview room is common among families of Heart Kids, or families of any gravely ill child. In a short corridor linking neonatal intensive care to its larger neighbour, the paediatric intensive care, was a side room, designated as an interview room. As we were ushered into the innocuous looking space, vague memory of the furnishings sprang to mind. The room had been redecorated by HeartKids NSW some years earlier, and I'd seen a photo online. The dark leather couches with their Chesterfield style buttons had been a dramatic advance on the flimsy, threadbare charmless seating that preceded them. The new chairs spoke of comfort and stability, conveying a sense of respect for the occupant. At the same time, the muted grandeur of the furnishings probably demanded more space, as they were packed tightly around the perimeter of the room. We each found seats, enjoying the dignity of physical comfort as we perched, and waited for the conversation we had to have.

Dimly, I recalled this room had served an earlier purpose in our life. Fourteen years ago, Maggie spent many hours ensconced either here, or in a room much like it, expressing breast milk, hoping our baby would survive to drink it. Around the corner and across the hall was a room where Malachy's first open heart surgery had been proposed and consented to, then later explained as a success.

A room just like this, on the other side of the city, was used to inform us on night one of Malachy's grand adventure of all the findings from his very first scans. In that room we had first endured the medical balancing act of hearing how bad were the problems we faced. Not only that, in that room we had also watched doctors search to find words to establish grounds for hope that the worst was not our fate.

The entwining dance of risk and hope, enacted in the secret sterile confines of a hospital interview room, had familiar rhythms.

The interview always begins without words. There is not silence, but the swinging of doors, people move close to enter then move apart to their respective seats. The seats creak or slide, according to their own constitution, or the qualities of the flooring.

The body language of the interview room is critical. Frank and direct eye contact tells of either good news or open questions: 'Your child is critical but stable', 'Technically, it is a good outcome, but we still have some hurdles to face'.

Brisk movement, ever the style of the optimist says: 'We still have treatments to offer', 'We are not done trying'.

Less eye contact, stiffening formality of movement: this is bad.

A wisp of gravitas, glances exchanged between the professionals conveys, 'We know something terrible', 'It's our job to tell them properly'.

Worst of all, damned if they do it, and worse if they don't, is the professional sad-eyed look of compassion. Doctors or nurses who seem to care for your child are for that time the most wonderful people in the world. When they look like they care about you, show compassion for the parent or sibling or loved one, there can be no good news.

We sat, a study in outward calm, and saw the glances.

I shifted in my seat and felt the edge of quiet, the gravitas.

Then I saw it in their eyes: compassion.

The trifecta.

So, we returned to the question of the day: 'Does an MRI show Malachy's brain is okay?'

No, it doesn't.

The best of medical evidence gathered for our benefit told us, at some point on day four, that, NO, there is no prospect the brain which has sustained your son and brother to rise above his limitations, can do so any longer.

I don't know what happens inside the heads of other people, or in whatever organ we suffer the enormity of love and loss. I don't know whether other people feel the same things I do, whether their chest seems it might burst even though there is nothing pressing on it, whether it seems, however briefly, that their life must just be ending, a shock of emptiness replacing whatever they had before. I was to have moments like this in the days following Malachy's return to the ICU.

When the silence of the interview room became filled with the rushing white noise of devastation, I felt my hand reach to my throat. I pressed on the top of my sternum. I didn't know what to do. I probably needed to scream in defiance of the tiny whisper-sized room, to yell at gods unknown and known, whether they existed or not. I probably needed to break things and blame people and cry and collapse. I clutched my chest and stayed, and asked more questions, and looked for unfounded hope. I felt my heart flutter and, in that instant, wondered if that was what Malachy felt, whether that was the warning he had before the ground of the school bus line broke his fall.

The dance would be repeated. We would agree to hear the news again from the neurologist, a woman of impeccable bedside skills, a sensitive tone and clarity of explanation. Even as part of my life ebbed away, and I hated where I was and what I was hearing, I knew these people were doing this well. They were skilful communicators and did all that could be done for a family in the throes of loss. Everything was done, and nothing could be done.

We would seek out our other children, and the dance would be replayed with them included. The worst of possible situations had the best of possible management.

'If he survives,' asked Imogen, frozen in her chair, not wanting to ask this, not wanting the answer, 'what will he be able to do?'

'The most likely situation, if Malachy does survive, is that he would be greatly disabled. He has suffered a severe brain injury affecting all parts of his brain,' said the doctor.

'So what about reading and talking?'

'It is not likely he will be able to communicate as he does now.'

Niamh, Seamus and Imogen wanted to know, 'What happens now?'

The doctor: 'We can continue to provide full intensive care and keep Malachy going as he is, or we can treat him to keep him comfortable. Do you think Malachy would want to survive if he cannot walk?'

'That depends. He is used to not being able to do things,' said Seamus.

'But if he can't think and talk...' Niamh tapered off. The sentence had nowhere to go.

Almost as one, the children conveyed, 'His brain is his life; if it's not working, he would not want to live'.

Doctor: 'After we withdraw support, we don't know how long it will take, but Malachy will die. We will be able to keep him comfortable.'

The round of interviews concluded at some point.

The dread that had stalked us at a greater or lesser distance, one child's entire lifespan was now made real. There was nothing left to fear.

We returned to Malachy's bedside.

50

SOUNDS OF FAREWELL

My Idea of Heaven Is… No arguing, fighting, poverty and murder. There would be no school and I'd be fourteen forever. Me and some other people would be extremely athletic, strong and fast.

— Malachy, May 28, 2010

Following our interviews, Malachy remained comatose, with death imminent and cure forsaken in favour of comfort; it was a different room we returned to. Malachy now required care of a sort rarely considered when we think of Intensive Care, the capital city of life-saving heroics.

What does death look like in this pale green ward dedicated to the pursuit of miracles of survival? We were amongst machines and people arrayed and trained to defy death, whatever the odds. Everything about ICU speaks of medical salvation.

It's crazy we don't recognise it, but of course people die with tragic frequency in Intensive Care Units. We had now entered a secret world in which special skills come to the fore. Officiousness can be useful when marshalling resources in the fight to live, but is unbearable in the presence of grief. No matter your level of competence, if you can't leave your ego at the door, you're no good to the dying.

The angels of mercy were summoned and sent into the fray. We needed them, the unheralded palliative 'A-Team'. The gifted comforters. Souls innately recognised as suited to dealing with death. People whose eyes speak of depth without judgment. People who convey unconditional concern for the movement of a family into mourning, and a child into permanent silence.

What little sound we made perched forlorn in the sterile single room echoed through the eerie quiet. Alarms and beeps were silenced, no longer required to demand urgent medical care. Futile medical care. A hollow dread replaced hope. How long could this last? How much would he suffer?

Despite so much silence ahead of Malachy, it seemed silence was all we could give him on this day. We had our verdict. Life was ebbing away. We were stunned into an eerie tearful vigil.

The worst day of my life had arrived.

The outside world still existed, we knew, because visitors came and went. We were comforted and in turn lent comfort to family and friends, leading them back and forward through the security door and up the barren hallway to Malachy's last hospital room.

The days dragged. Personal comfort was disregarded as Malachy's life, recently thought to be in its early days, was brought into focus as a completed package, a race run to its finish.

In the little time we had to come to terms with what was happening we had to grill the doctors, time and again, needing certainty that they were right; that the life inside our sleeping son and brother was truly extinct, that he was not in pain, that he knew nothing of his suffering. That there was no mistake. That we had to let him go.

Tenderness was all I could offer my son now, the beautiful would-be man who would no longer hear my jokes or join the banter. His needs were simple.

I looked to Maggie, slightly hunched, shoulders drawn up as if this posture of comfort could defeat the distress of the moment. Red-rimmed eyes fixed on her son's supine form, wedged onto an angle to prevent bed sores. As I watched, Maggie's blue-red eyes turned in the direction of the other children and I saw a movement. A lurch. A jolt. A scarcely perceptible shock of emotion as she spotted each child in turn. I saw this because I feared for her.

It is a parent's fate to fear what their child will suffer. Both Maggie and I saw the certainty of their brother's love torn from them on the cusp of adult life. All three would now leave their precious brother behind. The omnipresent ray of light that ran through their childhood was deserting them as we looked on, spectators to a drama we could not alter.

Ignatian ideas had been a source of inner strength for Maggie and me in the past, but now we were beyond our capacity for any kind of strength. With Malachy's death inevitable, no amount of indifference could make our situation bearable. We couldn't bear it bravely, or frantically, or any other way. We were discovering there is nowhere to turn when even the God of Good Outcomes lies dead in a roadside ditch.

Imogen rarely asserted any needs of her own through the 19 years we'd shared with her, but now stepped up.

'We can't leave him. One of us must be here all the time. If there is any chance he can hear anything, or feel anything, he can't be alone.'

If there were any rational chance he could perceive his surrounds, Imogen's roster would ensure he would perceive at least one of us there, with him. I urged Imogen to remember to sleep and eat, as we didn't know how long we'd have to endure.

'I can't; he needs to have someone here.'

The vigil was long. Malachy was never alone.

Maggie's eyes softened with water as her gaze struck Seamus, with another tiny shudder. Seamus was always a bit hard to read, something of a dark silent type, but with a mainline to parental heartstrings. Even as an infant, when upset, his distress was so heartfelt it dragged you in, so that you felt a piece of what you imagined he was experiencing. At that bedside in ICU his quiet was now impenetrable. Indecipherable emotion weighed heavily, but found no words, nor actions to name itself. Head bowed, glistening eyes, fingers rounded, clasping the nearest part of his dying companion. He'd said nothing and asked for nothing.

'Seamus,' Maggie uttered softly, 'would you like some time alone with Malachy?'

'Yes,' came the immediate response.

The rest of us left. Seamus and Malachy disappeared one more time into their private world where talk was hardly needed.

Niamh's relationship to Malachy had always been playful. Early in the hospital stay she had brought her sense of fun and life to the bedside, constructing a series of photos with Malachy and his toys. When he awoke, Mac would be entertained with a pictorial story in which two favourite toys make a stop-motion journey from his feet to a celebration tucked either side of his sleeping head.

'I feel bad now,' she said, 'that we joked with Malachy when he was dying, but I thought he'd wake up'.

'We all did, Niamh. It's okay.'

Who knows whether it's okay to have fun when your brother is dying? There is no rulebook.

We wanted this time to last forever, for us, the time we would have Malachy in our lives. For Malachy, we wanted the time to end.

No matter how much the medical evidence tells you, 'He feels nothing', a restless whispering voice in every vacant space says, 'End this pointless suffering.'

Into this unrelenting sombre atmosphere strode one of the doctors, and in a touching moment, granted us a permission we'd been too shell-shocked to grant ourselves.

'It's pretty quiet in here. Why don't you play some music or something? Do you have any music with you?'

Maggie replied, 'Actually we do'.

One of Niamh's old friends had brought a gift for Malachy, with whom she shared interest in a much-awaited new album from the Arctic Monkeys. 'We have a CD, but we don't have anything to play it on.'

'We can get you a CD player'

'That would be great.' We needed to do something about the pall that had descended, if not for us, then it may not be rational, but we could spark up for Malachy.

The disc went into the portable sound system. As the first stark jangling chords of Track 1, *Do I Wanna Know* burst from the stereo we all felt a jarring recognition, not only 'Yes, this is great' but also 'Malachy would be loving this'.

In a collision of art and life, the opening track was already a favourite of Malachy's, the enticing single that had been released a few months earlier. The promise of the album took until now to deliver.

Months later, Maggie would write in a letter about this day:

The Artic Monkeys,
Best Band in the World.

Dear Alex, Jamie, Nick and Matt,
This is an extraordinarily difficult letter to write. Please bear with me as I describe my special request of you at your Tuesday Sydney concert May 7th.
I am the proud mother of a very special 14-year-old boy who died last September. He was a mad, crazy Artic Monkeys fan as are his brother Seamus and sisters Imogen and Niamh. We are all coming to your concert and so too are many of Malachy's close friends in part as a special tribute to him but also because we are genuinely fanatical about you and your fabulous music.
Malachy Frawley was counting down the days to the September 6th release of AM last year with excited anticipation, making regular Facebook posts to all his friends and creating general over-the-top excitement. Unfortunately for us all Malachy collapsed from a massive heart attack at the school bus line on his way home from school on Tuesday 3rd of September and never regained consciousness dying in hospital on September 9th.
When we were delivered the devastating news that Malachy was severely brain damaged and the prospect of him dying was very likely many friends came to visit us as we sat by his bedside in ICU. One special friend bought a copy of AM for Malachy to listen to. The last 24 hours when we knew he was dying were extremely tense and at one stage the intensive care specialist doctor suggested we play some music to help our family to relax a little...

The music had echoed its way around the room, bouncing off the bland furnishings, the dull colourless indecorous walls and blinds and the cold of the glass partitions. Along the way it resonated. We were in the moment, and I had a sense that I knew Malachy would approve, would love the music, and would want us to enjoy it. Whatever complex emotions lay beneath, something good entered the room. We danced and the mood lightened. Track 2, *Are You Mine*, had been released as a single in early 2012. It had spent more than a year with pride of place in our music collection, helping build the anticipation for this album. It rang through the room with urgent intensity. I relived in an instant every moment I'd shared the joy of this riff with Malachy.

After the familiar thrills of the opening tracks, the album was all new and unfamiliar. But resonant. There would be months, maybe years ahead to wish we could share this with Malachy, and to wonder how much joy he'd have had listening to this long-awaited treasure, but for now all we had was the strange guilty pleasure of feeling touched by these sounds as we desperately strove to hold back the sadness of the moment. I am sure we enjoyed it more than sanity would permit. As Maggie would describe it:

... We played Malachy AM (several times) as he lay there in a coma, and I now have such a strong emotional attachment to this album as we have been playing it constantly since Malachy's death. The songs on this album all make me cry every time I hear them and they will be a living memory of watching my son die.

My request to you is could you please dedicate one of your songs to Malachy's memory during the concert. It would be an amazing gift to us as a family and to his friends who will be there. Any song, it doesn't matter as he loved them all. Just for you to mention his name on stage would be a lasting memory and an amazing gift to us.

I am going to keep this brief in the hope you read it.

Many kind regards,
Maggie Frawley

The unrelenting mournful quiet of that endless day in that bland hospital room gave way to a more demonstrative period in which Malachy was held and cried over, in which we said to him the things we needed to say.

51

MORE HUGS

We do survive every moment, after all, except the last one.

— John Updike

I wish I had not lived through those seven long days that September. I wish I could take them back and have them again, with a different outcome.

Those days are built of countless moments that live in memory.

Friends came and went. Malachy's friends, loved all the more by us for their devotion to our fragile son. These friends, so treasured by me for the joy they brought Malachy, stepped to the bedside one by one and said their piece, each in keeping with their experience of Mac.

'Mac, I have only known you for a short time, but already I feel that you are my best friend.'

'Mac, you are the bravest person I know, I know you will be with us and we will make you proud of your friends.'

'Mac, I will miss our arguments and discussions; it won't be the same...'

And so on.

His close friend PJ, with whom he shared innumerable hours and a love of literature sat by his bed and read to Malachy. This was another new release Malachy had sweated on, the latest novel from Rick Riordan, of 'Percy Jackson' fame. We gave them space while PJ read on, page after page, sharing one more time the excited admiration of someone's writing genius.

Ryan, who had been Malachy's closest ally at school since day one, ignoring and sharing in the invalid's social exclusion, was visibly shaken as he spoke to, and of, his friend in the dark knowledge that what they shared was ending.

Meanwhile, Malachy's heart beat on soundly, not a hint of the catastrophic pause in activity that had brought us to this pass. I strained against the ridiculous irony. Damn this stupid heart, which beats as if nothing has happened. Its perfect rhythm seemed to laugh in our faces. This is what it should have done five days ago.

As I watched his still, comatose body, a flicker of movement caught my eye. The muscle relaxant medication, so essential to the intubated patient, had worn off, making movement possible—if, of course, he could move.

There it was again, unmistakably, a twitch of the shoulder.

The pulsing in my chest increased. I felt it reach to my head. Though I knew the game was up, clearly, we humans are wired for hope.

The twitch became a jerk, and grew more frequent. Malachy's shoulder pulled forward; his head tugged sideways. I held his arm and wished stillness upon him. The jerks continued, stronger, more sudden. I felt his joints grind and begged the nurses and doctors to relieve the distress. Somewhere deep inside I couldn't be convinced the wrenching spasms did not trouble Malachy. I urged and questioned. Comfort was the goal of management, so if Malachy needs pain relief, how are we to measure his pain? If nothing hurts does he even need morphine?

The jerks bothered me. I hated them then as I do now. On and on the spasm of those muscles reminded me Malachy's brain was not in control. Some primitive fitting reflex had taken over.

'Please,' I asked, 'can we consider these jerks a sign of pain? Can we give him enough medication to calm this fitting?'

Sedatives and morphine would calm him for a time. I felt he needed more, though the expert doctors assured me the studies show the doses Malachy was having made pain impossible. We needed this to be true, because it looked awful.

We reached the limits of how much palliation the doctors believed they could ethically, legally provide. The guilty heart beat on. Malachy knew nothing, had spent days without any sign of consciousness or voluntary action. All that was left was for him to die, officially.

The brain could do nothing. The law allowed no active steps to stop the other functions from mindlessly ticking on. The shoulders jerked and the lungs rose and fell. Nobody could say how long this would continue.

We had always believed our son to be frail and been frightened to put pressure on his chest. For too many hours it seemed we underestimated the resilience of his vital core.

Care was needed. Lying frozen in bed day after day causes pressure. The skin breaks down if you don't move or be moved. Sweat and oils build up if not washed away.

I watched as a nurse gently, carefully tended my son. Noticing how intently we watched her go about her caring work, she extended the invitation to us to help. What else could we offer? I took a wet cloth and started on Malachy's face, gently wiping away the day's grime, sending as much love as I could through the palms of my hands, placing strands of hair just so—Mac would have wanted his coolness intact.

When the time came to wash Malachy's back the nurse indicated we should roll him towards us, onto his left side, allowing her firstly to clean the exposed skin, and to massage the potential points of pressure, preventing sores. The roll onto the side was also essential for the deft change of sheets. Somehow, I remain impressed by the nifty execution of this unheralded aspect of nursing teamwork. The grimy leftovers of a day's intensive care are whipped out from under the immobile hulk of a critically ill body, leaving it apparently undisturbed on crisp new linen.

With guidance from two nurses, the family took part in the roll. I was at the head end, at Mac's right shoulder, and shifted his arm a little to help achieve the required posture as his warm chest was eased upwards off the bed. Controlling his head to avoid neck injury I stooped low and held him close. His back was warm, the skin soft as I clutched him to me. His usually cyanosed skin was deepening in colour, faintly mottled from the pressure of the mattress, and the fading of his circulation. I held his chest to mine. I felt a soft rattle in his breathing as some secretions struggled to clear from his airway. There was at first a comforting calm rhythm to his breath, as I held him to me, as much to savour his embrace as to aid in the bathing routine. Then, out of the blue he stopped. A silent pause as the air expelled. Silence hung ever so briefly then breath resumed as I looked to Maggie. Had she felt it too?

For that moment it seemed a brief pause could become the last pause. Is that what death is? Merely a pause that continues as all previous like moments did not.

Death, the final pause, was clearly Malachy's goal now, clearly better than the living death of a useless globally impaired brain propped up by breath and heartbeat. A brain that allowed the repeated jerking of limbs, but no speech, no touch, no last familial eye contact, no meaning.

What purpose would be served by more waiting? We waited for those support organs to agree with the diagnosis. The heart needed to recognise the game was over. There was no living brain to perfuse. Blind and mute it beat on. Heedless, Malachy's chest rose and fell, as his lungs continued to drag in and push out once life-giving air.

Between the scheduled routines of personal care, we wept on Malachy and hugged him. We consoled each other, and our visitors, tried to eat, sometimes to sleep. On went the vigil as we each poured our love into the closing act of Malachy's life.

At one point I used my mobile phone to take the grainy photo that is pinned to the corkboard beside my desk. Malachy's stiff body and the hospital bed form the backdrop. The picture is taken from above, looking down. Meeting in the centre of the image are six hands piled one on the other, Malachy's topmost, with a lead running from his fingertip. The oxygen level is still being measured. Six recognisable arms fan out to the border of the image. All of us, the whole family, alive together. Or at least still sharing the warmth of living human flesh. Solidarity.

Malachy in hindsight had been gone for six days, but his body still needed our care.

After the momentary pause in breathing, I felt sure his condition was now fragile. I hoped it was fragile enough to release him, to guarantee the absence of all possible suffering. For now, we had only medical evidence to assure us he was untroubled. Proof would only be delivered one way.

I found myself hoping each episode of bathing or sheet changing, each physical turn would be the one that delivered our proof. The one to help Malachy across the River Styx, into Hades. It is likely the Greek version was his preferred take on what lies hereafter. Each chance to help with Malachy's comfort brought a sense of moment, a shimmer of hope we could help with his most pressing, final need.

I drew Malachy to me once more as part of his wash. Bringing his chest close to mine I felt my arms draw in as the air left his body, then drift out again as the warm pressure of his chest once more expanded. My fingers supported his narrow ribs, my wrist crossed the bony knobs of his spine, and his warm breath rustled at my neck. I held him closer as he breathed out, squeezing and relaxing ever so lightly, synchronised with his innate life-sustaining movement. Malachy's chest wall beat against mine as one long breath left past my shoulder, then stopped.

Unflinching, we waited for the next intake of air. Maggie's gaze met mine as I nodded minutely. We knew. We shared calmly the moment fourteen years dreaded, three days desired.

We waited.

When that breath didn't come the crying started.

MALACHY'S MAGNUM OPUS

Esteban Devereaux's Adventure

Chapter Three

— Malachy Frawley 2013

When Esteban awoke he couldn't figure out where he was. He eventually came to the conclusion that he was in a hospital.

These are the last words of an incomplete work.

PART 5

GRIEF

the shape of loss

52

RITUALS

For thousands of years we did have death surrounding us, and we did have people die in the home. You would take care of your own end. You would do ritual processes...

— Caitlin Doughty

Once Malachy had stopped breathing, his life was officially declared extinct and his death certified appropriately. Given the amount of information available prior to his final technical demise an autopsy was not likely to prove helpful to anyone.

Tentatively, a nurse raised with us some of the questions around the topic 'So What Happens Now'. We responded to an ill-defined feeling, half articulated, that nothing much can be any consolation, but you better try, just in case it matters later.

The tools of some secret ICU rituals included some potential options to mark Malachy's bodily departure. A set of translucent silk bags with decorative drawstrings were offered. In these we placed half-a-dozen locks of Malachy's flowing loose curls, carefully cut from the thicket at the back of his head. This was a previously undiscovered use of the nurse's ubiquitous scissors. The hair at the front would be needed intact for viewing in his casket. We had to exercise this small vanity on Malachy's behalf.

Time was not a problem, to a point, as we were told we could spend as long as we liked with Malachy. A risky offer to a family who never want to lose their child.

Paints and canvasses were shown to us, for the only opportunity to capture a handprint or footprint of the dead man. A chance to make a creative physical record of Malachy.

In our culture, so afraid of and ignorant of death this was all unexpected and unknown. Awkwardness attended every new aspect of the dialogue as we realised we had no cultural rules to fall in behind. I'd seen ritual painting on the bodies of the dead before. My job as a General Practitioner includes certifying the death of patients. I had learnt on professional visits to the mortuary of the beautiful traditional send off some Indigenous people give their beloved when I had pulled back a cover and found little patterns dotting significant parts of the face, limbs and body. The offer of paints for Malachy was outside of any such ritual framework. It appealed to our yearning to retain something of Malachy whose permanent absence had just begun.

In the end we took several bright-coloured imprints of both hands and feet, pressing his now cold, limp but gradually stiffening digits against the pliant white material. Left behind were the last physical traces, distinguished as his by our discerning eyes, noting the subtle expanse of Malachy's domes of finger clubbing where other fingers would taper.

His near-naked body, with a small blanket as modesty draping, would be bestowed with as much dignity as we could rally to the cause. After a thorough wash we dressed him in a favourite pair of jeans and a T-Shirt. A hint of blue residue from the paints couldn't be fully expunged and would stay with Malachy until his cremation.

Malachy would make his way separately back to Nowra, after the medical referee signed off on his appropriate certification, but not until we had finished our farewell. In the absence of circulation, Malachy now was pale, this time truly the colour of 'crossing over' as he had once laughed. Not only pale, but cold. So cold as I kissed his forehead and cradled either side of his head in my hands, that the diagnosis was confirmed by the lingering coolness on my lips and fingers. While a mind plays tricks and quibbles, the sensory evidence of death would not be denied. Death had really happened here.

A handful of futile tears were shed, and we left the room. As with the shock of any sudden event we could but wander back into the light of the sparse hospital hallways, stunned, unprepared for whatever this change meant to the rest of our lives. The drive home would be the first time we would know that feeling of vast emptiness. The whole living family present, incomplete.

The steel-blue Kia Carnival, bought for the family scale of its seating, and with Malachy's approval for the sound system, with its extra speakers adjacent to his third-row seat, now had no one to occupy that third row.

The world we returned to seemed suddenly full of experts in death, as we were guided through the public rituals with compassion and skill in variable proportions, by priests and funeral directors, friends and family.

There wasn't so much a comforting rhythm to ease us through the gap between death and burial, as a tide of collective activity. People too many to name stepped forward and removed from us the numerous burdens of necessary organisation. Our role was to be swept along, stopping at intervals to approve or tailor their actions.

As parish priest and longstanding pillar of the Nowra community, Father Pat Faherty, was faultless in his pastoral care and counsel. His assistant, Father Duane, a friend to Malachy and much liked by all of us, had the daunting task of delivering a homily at the funeral. This would be the biggest liturgical event to that point in his still brief career as a priest, made all the more challenging by his personal closeness to Malachy.

The school communities of St Michael's and St John's swept into action on the service, the booklets, the music, even raising a choir for the event. This was dovetailed in with the beautiful work by some of our friends leading the music, which did justice to the lost life. Maggie's family were on hand, especially her sister Tess, to run cover domestically, taking charge of phones and doors, and even somewhat beyond the brief, acquiring new plants for the garden.

People asked me while I pondered the task ahead whether I would be capable of speaking at my own son's funeral. I was more inclined to think it would be impossible for me not to speak, deprived as I was of any ability to do anything more for the treasured life I mourned. Honouring Malachy in some way was all I had left to give him.

The famous anthropologist, Bronislaw Malinowski, studied the use of rituals in South Pacific Islander communities. One of his observations was that people were more likely to undertake rituals when they faced uncertainty, threat and loss of control. Fishing in shark-infested ocean beds would be preceded by elaborate rituals, seeking magical protection, while fishing in protected waters involved no preparation of note. Whether you believe in such invoked powers or not, rituals give a structure to your grieving. Two people by the names Gino and Norton, researching the effect of rituals, reported in the *Scientific American* in 2013 evidence that 'Rituals appear to benefit even people who claim not to believe that rituals work'. Irrespective of utility, I was grateful for the structure.

One thing we chose in those dark days between death and cremation was to have Malachy on display, his casket open, at the funeral parlour. Maggie had taken Seamus shopping in the main street to help find a new suit for his dead brother. Malachy's love of suits helped us feel we knew how he'd like to be displayed in his last moments. Viewing Malachy in public, with his life extinct, was either unappealing to Maggie, or beyond her ability in the immediate throes of our grief. I wanted to see him, to be in his company once more, to tell him I don't know what.

The children and I didn't speak on the short drive down. The building rose from the street with the undertaker's typical eerie subdued formality. Once inside the décor, too, matched the stereotype, working so hard at being unobtrusive as to announce its purpose blatantly. We were directed to a side chapel, opening

285

the door into a room, with a dozen rows of chairs, nearly empty of people. Music played softly, while gentle western sun filtered through stained glass, a rainbow of colour falling across the front of the room.

The rainbow cast its glow on a white box in a front altar section. From the doorway I saw the lid of the box had been removed. Emptiness and fear combined. Seeing Malachy here wouldn't make him any more dead, or bring him any closer to life, but would give vivid proof, visual confirmation of all that I didn't want to believe.

We sat for a while, so caught in the heady emotions of the time I am no longer sure who else was there. I think his closest friends, PJ and Ryan, were with us, Ryan's parents, then I'm not sure. People took turns walking to the front, seeing what they needed, and returning to sit. I approached both for myself and to support those who faltered or needed a living hand or arm in support.

Malachy's face was serene, the colour adjusted skilfully to mimic his living image. His skin was cold, refrigeration cold, with only that faint blemish on his right upper eyelid to betray the torture of his week of dying.

His suit—perfect. Proudly 'suited up' would be the style of his leaving.

Malachy's flowing hair, its many hues of colour undiminished in death, was combed back from his brow, a small departure from his usual style of attentive messiness. I reached down to 'fix' this, finding the quiff stiff with hair product, and resolved to accept that a touch of mafia-styling was locked in. Malachy, had he known, may have enjoyed the theatricality of departing as a 'Don'.

Looking down at the detail of his sharp-dressed body I noted the care with which his hands had been prepared, resting prone at the top of his pin-striped thighs, tilted toward each other, a position of rest. The left hand swollen, a deeper blue than its neighbour, having borne the brunt of the last days of fluid therapy, which leaked into the tissues as his circulation failed. Part of me hoped this bloated trace of failed medical intervention would have been painted away in the back room. Seeing the size of the fingers I knew this hope to have been forlorn. A picture of serenity, with harsh truth hidden in the fine detail.

Uselessly pouring my love into him with my gaze, I said whatever I said, and shed whatever tears. Tears had become unnoticed by their repetition. Unable to leave his room, I returned to my seat, noticing as I turned two more people in the room. Camille and her mother. Minutes passed while I sat in contemplation. It dawned on me the young woman had not taken the path to the casket, and I wondered whether permission was needed, whether our distraught row of family may prevent other mourners claiming their emotional stake in Malachy. Unable to know what she and Malachy imagined for the future of their friendship, it struck me that a ritual farewell might have some value. I chaperoned Camille to the casket.

Who knows?

Once everyone had left, except for me and the four Frawley children, we took some photos, for Maggie and for our grief. How similar to himself in life he looks in those photos, but how different it feels to look on those images and to know the lights were out.

The myriad of necessary preparations for a funeral service ticked along, as we nervously hoped we were missing nothing. Of course, we missed some things, but, heh, did anything matter anymore?

In terms of ritual, after the viewing all that was left was the funeral, the last hoorah.

We had to survive to and through Malachy's funeral and wake.

53

SAYING GOODBYE

Meantime the hellish tattoo of the heart increased. It grew
quicker and quicker, and louder and louder every instant.

— Edgar Allan Poe, 'The Tell-Tale Heart'

I lay on the bed and counted, while my heart raced within the
cage of my chest. I tried to be still, and calm, and patient. One
hundred and forty beats per minute, I counted. That's twice my
usual speed. It made me feel weak and a touch light-headed.

In one hour's time I was expected to climb the stairs to the stage
of the school hall to deliver a eulogy for Malachy. That was going to
be physically difficult if my heartbeat wouldn't get back to normal.

It seemed the world should stop, that life as we knew it had
ended, but instead it now spun faster. As I lay nervously distressed
everything raced. I tried to rest but the roar of the world changing
speed was simply too loud.

Clutching my wrist at intervals, I felt for the tapping insistence
of my radial artery, so often used to tell life from death. Searching
for that spot in the groove above the bone I sought in vain for the
reassurance I was back in a normal rhythm. Public speaking was
not my forte at the best of times and this persistent tachycardia
seemed a recipe for panic, until all of a sudden it stopped. With ten
minutes to spare, I was suddenly, unexpectedly still and ready.

My effusive brother-in-law, Bill, always willing to shoulder a
load for anyone in need, took on the task of driving the immediate

family to the funeral, one block away. Desperate for quiet, and anticipating Bill's insistent murmurs of encouragement, we had Tess, his wife, issue him an order to say nothing en route.

Malachy's farewell being too big to fit in St Michael's church, it had been moved to the nearby school hall. Our friends in the band had the evocative strains of Coldplay's 'Yellow' filling the vast space of the hall, echoing into the adjoining playground as we entered by a side door. Under the melodic din of the music was a palpable hush, as those who had already gathered in the hall noticed our arrival. A jolt of recognition passed through me as I saw the coffin. The moment became real.

Adopting the vacant seats front and centre, we then went forward to the coffin, each with a symbolic gift for our dead son and brother. The stark white coffin was being steadily adorned with texta messages, as arrivals queued to leave a mark of their love for the young man inside.

In blue texta: *Dear Malachy, You were the strongest person I ever knew... You will be forever missed.*

In black: *Malachy, One of the happiest, funny and strongest people...*

In red: *Malachy you will be loved and missed by all. You're in my heart forever, Swag Monster.*

Red again: *From your Fav Yr11, We love you and miss you, Mal Dog.*

In blue: *We'll miss you my main man. Hope we weren't as important to you as you were to us.*

All the available space was covered with professions of love, little private jokes he'd shared with the writers, anecdotes of their contact with the person inside the box, thoughts that would later be turned to heat and ash, along with the body inside.

It seemed we'd barely taken our seats when the order of service found me called to address the congregation. Somewhere my mind found time to wonder what it would be like to die unmourned, as it dawned on me how many people were assembled. The crowd filled the hall, and spilt onto the courtyard behind, and the playground beyond that. Speakers had been placed outside to accommodate the numerous mourners who couldn't be squeezed inside.

After ascending to the podium, against the accumulated weight of collective grief and silence, I faced the microphone. Looking out across the hall, the coffin level with my feet in the centre aisle and every face turned to me, initially stunned by the scale of the crowd, I fumbled the opening lines, skipping a stanza before backtracking with an apology and an embarrassed smile. The gentle murmur from the congregation stated the bleeding obvious—that I would never have a more sympathetic audience.

Inspired by the countless happy memories of Malachy's life, of his humour, and his generous nature, a curious joy found voice that day. A single flower bloomed in a terrible wasteland. Malachy ignoring the finality of death, inspired me from the casket.

> I am up here to talk to you about a man like no other, a charmer without peer and a profound philosophical prodigy; a child who didn't recognise the false barriers of age, gender, or race, an upstart who really didn't know his place.
>
> This 'boy who lived' has given me a difficult brief. His request as described to Maggie was: 'Tell Dad, at my funeral I want him to crack some gags. I want people to laugh at my funeral.'

I spoke of Mac's place in our family.

> Clearly Mac's effect on our family was dramatic from the start, and his siblings' lives took on a shape that not only accommodated, but then encouraged and exaggerated his penchant for colour, drama and humour. He was putty in the hands of Imogen, Seamus and Niamh, who teamed up to manhandle him, tease him, challenge him, and the return they have had is a lifetime of love, and of laughter which makes Malachy so easy to mourn. Laughter was his constant companion.

Emboldened by the urge to honour Malachy and mindful of his fanciful imagination, I strove to include some of the mandated humorous touch:

> He had some difficulty distinguishing his imaginary life from his actual one, or his favourite books from the daily news. Once the Harry Potter phenomenon took hold (in our home) Malachy would act out entire 'cast of thousands' scenes solo. Including one lively day the Troll scene from The Philosopher's Stone. The climax of the scene saw Mac acting both the troll and Harry, as our hero rammed his wand into the nose of the giant intruder who crashed to the ground defeated. Intent on realistic action, Malachy (as Harry) used a pick-up stick rammed into the nostril of Malachy (the troll) as he fell to the lounge room floor. When I heard Maggie's shrieking, I rushed to find a scene of disaster, Malachy, pick-up stick lodged six inches into his nose, hosing blood all over himself and the room. He sure taught that troll a lesson.

I ended up summarising what I felt to be the essence of the moment:

> Malachy was a source of generous love towards so many people. I honestly could talk all day about wonderful and caring things he has done for people we might have thought were less needy than him. The beautiful and funny moments, the memory of his wit and vibrancy, his suits and ties, and so many other things have sustained us through this week and will sit astride any sadness we feel. We will live on proud to carry him in our hearts for eternity.
>
> Malachy, with courage and grace you have built your ladder to the stars, now my friend you can rest, and stay forever young.

I walked back down the stairs from the stage and resumed my seat beside the coffin.

Following the template of the mass, some sacred texts were read before the baton was passed to Malachy's friend and mentor, Father

Duane. Malachy was a great admirer of Duane, and for good reason. They had come to know each other quite well, making Duane the only choice for the task that now fell to him. For the first time as priest Duane would perform the homily for a friend, to the largest congregation of his nascent clerical career. In his naturally modest, gentle tone, he began like this:

> It's hard for me to imagine what it would have been like for Malachy, growing up with so many limitations that he knew other kids his own age didn't have to deal with.
>
> It's even harder to imagine how he managed to face these limitations with such uncomplaining patience and courage, with such a self-forgetful generosity of spirit even from a young age.
>
> How was it possible that in the midst of all his limitations he was able to brighten up our lives so much with his wonderfully quirky sense of humour, reflected for instance in 'D-money's account of Mac's upbringing, and of course his YouTube videos which hopefully will go viral any day now.
>
> How was it possible that in March this year on the morning of a major heart operation, his main concern when I met with him and his parents was not about himself, but about how his parents would cope with having to worry about him during the operation.
>
> How was it possible that one so young had such a deep passion for social justice; such a deep desire to make the world a better place, a place of peace and justice for all.
>
> In short: how did one so young touch so many people so deeply, in so short a time?

He knew Malachy and read him well. I didn't know of those privileged moments he described, with my son worrying for me behind my back, but it rang true. Too many times I have been to funerals and felt hollow proclamations of the 'deep faith' of the departed. To me that has become code for 'I scarcely know the deceased, but they did go to mass...' Even in the haze of grief I remember feeling relieved at the accuracy and honesty of Duane's words.

He went on to make sense of personal faith in a way that could comfort believers without grave offence to adherents of science and reason. His framework placed Malachy at peace, without the triumphal blather of 'Eternal Life' and 'Right Hand of the Father' talk. Such talk always strikes me as much less useful than having the cherished person alive.

Duane spoke of his belief in a God who loves Malachy as his own child and would welcome him to another life, and tied the idea in with a true sense of Malachy's own nature, as a person who wanted to improve the world he lived in:

> Malachy was longing for a place where there was no more suffering or sadness, where peace, and love and justice were at home. And it's into that place that we are letting Malachy go. Where at last Malachy will find the fulfilment of his deepest longings.
>
> And heaven is not some distant place unconnected with us. Heaven is always close to us, as we remember in a special way at every Mass. And in every Mass, when we pray as Jesus taught, your will be done on earth, as it is in heaven, we remember that we should all be longing for heaven, AND that this longing should lead us all to passionately seek to do our little bit to bring a little more of heaven to earth.
>
> This is what Malachy did, during his time with us. Malachy, 'messenger of God', brought a little bit more of heaven to earth.

Comforting tones of ancient Catholic prayers took us through a ritual rise and fall, the time disappearing in a blur of familiar incantations and beautiful heartfelt music, until the ceremony finished.

Several men who had borne Malachy for some part of his life now bore him again in death. Our heedless tears were met with a parting of the crowd, as the decorated coffin made its way to a hearse. Blessings were cast over Malachy, with ritual splashes of holy water. One minutely remembered moment I would rather forget followed another through the day. We drove past a guard of honour. Balloons were set free. People cried with us and for us. Malachy was cremated out of town at the lawn cemetery, with family at hand. We returned to his wake.

The celebration of Malachy's life was held across the road from home, in the local Showground. A heady blend of faces and personalities from umpteen phases of our life crowded together in a marquee and adjoining community hall, spilling in clusters into the surrounding grounds. We all had a share of the familiar view from Hanging Rock, looking west along the Shoalhaven River.

Schoolfriends, work friends, HeartKids colleagues at arms, Nowra locals and people from far-flung towns engaged us with ardent goodwill. The recurring joy of greeting old friends was constantly stalked by the sombre reality that drew them to the place. What is the correct way to feel when the death of your child brings old friends back into view? It was like a joyous wedding stacked with reunions, with an unwritten rule 'Guests must remember: Do Not Be Happy'.

We feasted and drank and talked. Music was played and photos and films were shown. It was a wonderful consolation to see and to be acknowledged and cared for by so many well-loved people. A permanent loyalty will endure towards all those who made our passage into life after Malachy so buoyant, so colourful and so well fed.

Sadness threatened to overwhelm me as I watched a group of Malachy's friends pose for the photographer, their lives to run on without him. One missing a confidante, one a peacemaker, while another lost a debating partner or a constant companion.

Talking at length to one friend or relative, meeting friends of Maggie's for the first time, or flashing back with my parents' friends from my childhood, I found myself ensconced outside the marquee, on the fringes of the melee. Departing guests shared their thoughts of Malachy or the arduous day now tapering to its conclusion.

Dad approached, his habitual posture proudly erect, with a tear reluctant to leave each eye. Placing a hand on my shoulder as others stepped back to allow him the moment, he looked at me. The weight of current sadness mingled with the other burdens of his 74 years, defied by his upright stance and erudite tone.

'You made me feel very proud today, Dominic, very proud.'

'Thanks, Dad.'

We exchanged some more commentary and Mum stepped forward for a hug, her hunched kyphotic stoop and shuffling gait a counterpoint to Dad's imperious bearing. More than 30 years beyond the crippling brain injury that sapped her of memory and language dexterity, Mum had no words at the ready to match the occasion.

'Dominic, darling,' she managed, clasping me. There would be many moments of sadness that cried out for maternal comfort in the months and years to follow. Those moments would confront me with the tyranny of circumstance—my mother's impaired communication, and the tyranny of distance—the downside of rural isolation from my family of origin.

Breakdown was not an option as my aging parents melded back into the throng and the cadence of greeting and farewell continued. As people made their presence known to me and offered their thoughts, more than one said words to this effect:

'I didn't meet Malachy, but after hearing you speak, I feel now I really know him.'

'It was lovely to get to know what Malachy was like.'

As it was when coping with the many shocks of Malachy's birth and early life, Maggie and I felt a responsibility to manage the grief of others. We understood that it falls innately to the bereaved family to set the tone.

Thus began the rest of my life.

54

EMPTY DAYS

I have not forgotten those who lost their sons when mere children;
but Cato lost his when full-grown with an assured reputation.

— A.C.Grayling, *The Good Book*,
Consolations, Chapter 1, Verse 16

My attention turned to the support of the surviving family
members. I wanted to take all their pain and carry it for
them. I wanted to be strong and steadfast and protect each of
them from what lay ahead. Anyone who has been clobbered by
grief knows it simply doesn't work like that. The world of pain
was all encompassing, both the shared pain of a family forever
now incomplete, and the individual worlds of personal loss.

A few weeks after the funeral, Maggie and I drove Niamh back
to resume the next term of boarding school. Term four of Year 10,
living with the girls she was just getting to know, having moved to
the school at the start of that year. Her new school friends had never
met Malachy. Not knowing how this may play out we decided to
take a hotel room in a nearby suburb and 'be there' for Niamh. The
plan was no clearer than that.

As we checked ourselves into the hotel and began the walk to
our room I felt as if a gloom had descended. The smiling staff
gave no sign that they'd noticed the obvious change, the inexorable
onward march of events. A rational voice inside must have stopped
me from returning to the counter to remind the staff, 'Don't you

know Malachy has died? The world has stopped. Make peace with yourselves and others. Nothing else matters.'

As we entered the room, and dropped our baggage, it wasn't so much, 'Nothing else matters' as, 'Nothing matters'. Hollowed by grief, barely going through the motions of this ordinary activity, Maggie slid open the doors to the courtyard beyond. We each looked briefly around the room as a breeze billowed a light synthetic curtain into the room. We cast an expressionless, knowing glance at each other, each climbed onto a side of the queen bed, lay back fully clothed, and cried. Wordlessly we sobbed as the light of mid-afternoon brightened, then dimmed. We gazed briefly out the open doors, where we could see beauty survived in theory. Then cried some more.

We made eye contact from time to time, understood our base human need, and cried some more, sometimes hand-in-hand, sometimes preferring the solitude of our own space on the bedcover. The constant sorrow and unrestrained tears were strangely calm. We understood as if by instinct these tears were normal. We knew nothing would stop them.

The irresistible power of grief sparked my curiosity. How could something with no rational use be so completely overwhelming? In the same way as we know nothing is ever solved by worrying, no one is resurrected by grief.

The only thing in the world I desired was to have Malachy back, with me, to see him live, to hear his jokes, and to feel dragged in by his enthusiasm. Unable to have what my heart desired, hormones and chemicals combined inside me to make water pour from my eyes. I remember commenting how strange and true it was that I was just a tiny organism, powerless to stop this chemical process of deep unbearable melancholy. Some natural poison in me forced this upon me, coming ready or not. Humans like to think we're beyond our animal ancestry, governing our emotions with reason.

Tell that to the grieving.

Mute animal distress would fill most moments of reverie for weeks and months to come.

In public appearances I may have appeared distant, distracted or flat, but the distraction of company did serve to suspend the competing themes of empty silence and wailing. The desperate hollow void could be occupied briefly. When all five of Malachy's surviving parents and siblings were together tears served no purpose. Inherently we all knew where we were at. Togetherness was my only pleasure.

To stop whatever was going on in my head, or my heart, or wherever the jangling chaos of grief is located, I found number puzzles some use. Sudoku brought me no joy, containing no intellectual challenge as such. The puzzles require only attention; keep focusing and take care with each step, and eventually you finish. This blocked all feeling for a time. While not being sure exactly what was bubbling away, vexing me, I knew it to be a calling card of grief, and to turn it off for the time it took to number a whole bunch of squares gave some respite. Each puzzle gave a small patch of stillness. As I filled the last number, the completion of each puzzle culminated in a resumption of the white noise of emotional pain.

More than two years later, my brain still seeks this masking agent in times of insomnia. No pleasure, but no noise.

Thinking about our loss had too many dead ends. The commonest, and worst form of dead end is the 'What If'.

Thinking 'What If' has a terrible gravitational pull for me. I try to stay away, intuiting the danger, like the edge of a black hole, or the more familiar giddy phobia drawing me off the edge of a cliff. I know 'What If?' is a terrible question that only causes pain, but it needles away; 'What if he hadn't missed any doses of aspirin?' 'What if we'd started some medication for the heaviness?' 'What if he'd called me at lunch time?' 'What if he'd just stopped running when he felt short of breath?' 'What if the teacher had noticed he wasn't right earlier in the day?'

On and on and on it could go. Each question has consequences. Each implies something could have been different. Each implies somebody could have done something, somewhere, to change the horrible trajectory of Malachy's death.

Maggie fell into the spiral of 'What Ifs' over and again, being less certain than me about avoiding the pain. Day after day her wounds reopened. While I had an intuition to avoid the fateful question, I had no adequate words to frame that advice for my wife.

A retired GP, a patient of mine, attended one day once I had dared venture back to work. He passed me a letter which he said may or may not apply, but contained his top grief tips from his years working in psychological medicine.

First and foremost, he advised, 'Avoid the What Ifs'. The timing was perfect, as Maggie perched on the edge of the vortex, the letter struck home with just enough force to help her into a steadying pattern. A mini salvation was effected by the rational eloquence of the right advice at the right time.

In the very early days, the five of us were at home one Monday evening, struggling to summon the will to self-care, thinking up a bland dinner to share, when the doorbell rang. One of the children proved brave and energetic enough to answer the door and returned up the hall with a beautiful two-course meal. A couple had dropped by, declining to 'interfere' with a visit, they had prepared and delivered a feast for the grieving family.

The next Monday, and the one after, it happened again. I don't know how many weeks this ritual of care and generosity was repeated.

Other people had the same idea, meals came in from all quarters. We were unable to avoid eating well. Our urge to self-neglect would have to find another form of expression!

I learnt a lot about how to help people in their time of need. So much, it made me realise I'd never properly learnt to care. If grief doesn't break me, I feel better armed to be useful in a future tragedy.

The hollowness of those early weeks and months after Malachy's death remains beyond description. So much of life passed by me unrecognised. Music washed over me, people came and went while a haze stayed with me.

I wanted to role-model appropriate help-seeking behaviour, so I booked myself into a visit to a psychologist. The woman I chose was known to me and had provided helpful care to many of my patients in the preceding years, but there was almost nothing she could do. This endless miasma of suffering was apparently normal. I say 'almost nothing' because something I couldn't do was work out how and when to resume working, so I implored the psychologist to tell me what to do. 'Don't rush' was her sage advice. Professional permission to keep grieving was somehow comforting.

The company and reflections of other parents who had lost children was like manna from heaven. Fairly or not, I entertained a prejudice that their insights were more valuable than that of others, many of whom were frank in stating they 'don't know what to say...'

A saddening current through all the darkest early days was all the life ahead that would no longer happen. It dawned on me ever more clearly just how much parental love is directed to the future you hope your child will have. Concern and effort are poured into education, to secure an as yet undefined career. Behaviours are refined and corrected to ensure social acceptability, and more than that, lovability. You want your child to be happy, in the future. Death makes it clear that future is illusory. Malachy's future, so profoundly mourned, so painfully lost, in fact never existed. His complete life ended after the first fourteen-and-one-half years. What I cry about so much was not Malachy's real life, but his imagined one.

Unfortunately, my imagined future had him in it. I have to live on without him. There will be no fireside chats, no comparing of essays, no debriefing about love lost or found, no challenge of learning to drive, or excitement taking possession of the keys to that first home. There will be no advice in time of crisis, nor joy in triumph, nor joking for the heck of it. All these things I have done with Malachy, many times in my mind, but never in life.

The dead person doesn't share these thoughts, nor feel this pain. They are gone.

So, in mourning, you cry for yourself.

Some people choose to read their way through grief—feel their way through the experiences of others. I didn't want that, having always preferred to discover my own path through life, but I did seek ideas. I did look to find as many ways to frame the conundrum of death as I could, knowing that I couldn't be the first to face what is a universal challenge, albeit exaggerated when the victim is your child.

Reason had long ago buried my childhood belief in an afterlife, once I found Bertrand Russell and friends vastly more cogent, compelling and persuasive than the combined teachings of millennia of religious scholars. Faith would have no power to console, but when push came to shove, I wanted to know whether secular wisdom could offer any help through what A.C. Grayling might call, 'the perennial challenge of being human'.

As it turned out, Grayling's *The Good Book* had drawn together the collected wisdom of humanity in a form that allowed me to find some solace. Ideas can be discovered and developed, but emotions will follow their own inexorable course. Feelings could not be tamed, but I wanted to review the ideas that would make satisfactory sense of Malachy's death. In any case it is likely I will have further grief in life, and inevitably a death of my own.

Malachy tended to trawl the world for ideas, in a youthful version of Grayling's search for wisdom. Grayling's tome, resulting from his hunt through history for human insights includes this verse, in which Laelius reflects on the death of Scipio:

> 21. To Scipio I am convinced no evil has
>   befallen. Mine is the disaster, if
>   disaster there be; and to be prostrated
>   by distress at one's own misfortunes

does not show that you love your
friend, but that you love yourself.[11]

While I knew nothing of the lives of either Laelius or Scipio, it
was comforting to know that other people had grappled with a loss
like mine and recorded their struggle, more than two thousand
years ago. It helped to be reminded my pain belonged to me, not
Malachy, whose ashes could not suffer, and knew nothing of his fate.

My suffering would however have the potential to harm others.
I had once had a friend describe to me the loss of his brother, setting
in motion a childhood in which, 'My mother cried at the dinner
table, every single night, from that day on. Every single night'.

Apollonius had lost his son, thousands of years earlier. He fell
into a funk of grief once the uncontrollable distress of the early days
had passed. A friend, acknowledging the severity of the prostrating
'unexpected calamity', went on to advise him:

21. Nothing is ever accomplished by
    yielding too far to grief and painful lamentation.
22. Now is the time for courage and
    endurance, now is the time to turn
    our thoughts to the living who are
    dear to us too,
23. And not to take ourselves from
    them, but to help them with our
    own patience and strength to bear
    what must be borne; for they bear
    it too.[12]

For better or worse, these insights rang true to me. So, the
instructions I took from these verses were: Malachy is okay, don't
worry about him. The others are still alive, be there for them.

Our surviving children each had very different ways of dealing
with their loss, which made it hard to know how to help them.

---

11 Consolations, 1:21
12 Consolations 3:21-23

They found grief very hard to talk about. Even the Good Book didn't answer all the questions their grief would pose.

Other angles the ancients tried by way of consolation included talk of the inevitability of death; you know it's coming, and we will all be ashes in the end, so cop this straight; it is reality. Or, nature and chance are fickle, if you're happy to accept the good luck that comes your way, you must also accept the bad.

Michael Leunig, the Australian cartoonist, had an alternative take on grief, shared with us by a friend rocked by the death of his gorgeous wife within months of Malachy's funeral. Stuck to our fridge door by a pair of magnets, amongst the tip vouchers, stray invitations and family photos is our copy of Leunig's offering, from 1980:

> When the heart
> is cut or cracked or broken
> do not clutch it.
> Let the wound lie open.

More than that, he recommends:

> … bathe the wound with salt
> and let it sting.[13]

If I had the capacity to choose, I could go with the stoic advice of our ancient forbears, to bear it silently, or adopt a more contemporary sensibility and wallow to the utmost. I couldn't count the number of people who I have heard over the years express the view that it is unhealthy, or even dangerous to 'bottle-up' your grief, that people MUST cry before they can move on. Leunig was making the most eloquent expression of this belief. I must say wallowing or stoicism each appealed in its own way. As month follows month I try each method, wallowing a while, then pushing it down. I watch the progress of my wife

---

13 Excerpts from Michael Leunig's poem, 'When the heart'.

and children, and know in my core this process will linger, its shape and shadow shifting with time.

Acute grief doesn't pause to allow a careful choice of technique. Nature charts the early course. Whether it is rational or not, our humanity is laid bare in the universal experience of grief. The trick seems to be in how you curtail the florid symptoms once that first storm ebbs. Lie low for the early storm, then launch your coping strategy.

Be warned, as Marcia was in ancient time, that the passing of the storm is not a forgone conclusion. Marcia's friend accused her of hugging and embracing '...the sorrow you have kept alive in place of this newly lost one', and lamented that:

> 8. Even time, nature's great healer, that
>   heals even our most grievous sorrows,
>   in your case has lost its power.
> 9. Three whole years have passed,
>   and yet the violence of your
>   sorrow has in no way abated.
> 10. Your grief is renewed and grows
>   stronger every day – by lingering it
>   has established its right to stay...[14]

Linger? Stay? This might go on for years? For ever?
    I didn't need to read that.

---

14 Consolations 6: 8-10.

55

MUSIC TO GRIEVE BY

Bad news comes, don't you worry even when it lands
Good news will work its way to all them plans

— Modest Mouse, *Float On*

In a small office beside a pontoon on the Huon River the young woman at the counter shrugged uncomfortably: 'I'm sorry, we don't seem to have your booking'.

Impotent in the face of bureaucratic confusion, I decided my goal was to be patient, let nothing break my calm. 'But I confirmed with you only yesterday, the name is Frawley, for five people'.

'I have a booking for six people.'

'Yes, that was my booking but we changed it to five.'

An older woman, probably the proprietor, was invited over to help sort our problem. Our Tasmania Attractions Pass was having technical problems.

'In our system it looks as if we are waiting on six people for the next tour.'

Patience wasn't a problem for me, it was something else that bothered me. The children peered through the window from the deck beyond, wondering, starting to raise their shoulders. I wanted to preserve the quizzical, 'What's the problem?' looks on their faces. The particular hold-up was becoming familiar.

Not wanting an audience, I leaned forward, and lowered my voice. 'You see, we made our booking a few months ago. Since then,'

305

I tried to avoid a perceptible pause, tried not to betray any emotion, 'since we made the original booking, my son has died. So there are no longer six people.'

The other customers waiting for attention pretended not to hear but kept enough distance to show they would not hassle just now.

'There are only five. There is no sixth person coming with us.'

'Bear with me.' Her response was inflected with kindness. It was the sort of saddened, kind response we were hoping not to deal with. Another unnecessary reminder of a pain we couldn't escape.

The five surviving Frawleys were on the road in Tasmania, on the run in the Malachy-endorsed Kia Carnival. Despite being a cumbersome vehicle with its very long wheelbase and a touchy accelerator, it was perfect for a trip planned for six. Now with only five of us its vast interior spoke of what was missing.

Driving the country lanes and highways of Tasmania, I tried to stay in the moment, to be mindful of our new, reduced family, and to enjoy all that we encountered. As usual, music was our companion on the road. Time and again a tune redolent of Malachy would crash through my defence, and I'd find tears pouring down my cheeks. They poured effortlessly, quietly, kept secret from the children in the back, I hoped. This was January, and we'd had four months of interminable sadness; I think we were all wanting it to end. Certainly, the youngsters were clear they wanted to start being happy again, to resume collecting good experiences.

Music was supposed to help, but the problem was Malachy. He'd invaded almost all the music. Malachy had an opinion on most bands, and he'd shared it with us. He had a passion for the stuff he liked, and again, we knew what that was. It seemed my wiring had been damaged, such that I only heard music through the filter of Malachy. A song he had loved was an acute reminder, as was the British Indie sound that we'd so enjoyed discussing and analysing. A song he hated, ditto. A band that sounded like the stuff he loved would make me want to know how he would have received it. 'This is such Malachy music' I would opine from time to time. The tears hadn't gone away as hoped. Anything sad—bang, they were back. Anything referring to death, loss, love, or family—bang, gone again. The Arctic Monkeys' 'AM' was of course on the playlist, with every track sending me plunging back to that anguished hospital room. Closer to Malachy, closer to the heart of my pain.

Okay, so I couldn't keep my ongoing sadness secret from the children. The Kia was big, but not that big. Instead, I would just find a way not to impose my sadness on them. Any periods of forgetful happiness anyone was capable of were well deserved by now.

Tasmania is a beautiful place to travel, with pristine waterways and forests, quaint heritage towns, uncrowded roads and numerous national parks. It is an Island offering outdoor activities to suit any grade of explorer. Mindful of Malachy's limitations we had carefully planned a trip full of the activities he was capable of. River cruises, short walks, some market-time in urban Hobart. We'd found one perfect option, in a park offering off-road Segway riding tours.

We had all had turns on Malachy's Segway. On a family holiday a couple of years earlier, at Samurai Beach, we had devised a Segway time-trial course around a tennis court complex and raced off against each other. By the time we enrolled for the forest tour outside Launceston, the whole family had become proficient at controlling the device.

After another hushed confirmation of the change from a six to a five-person booking, we undertook our safety instruction, strapped on helmets, and mounted our Segways.

My feet gripped the plates, and instantly I was back on Malachy-time. It had always felt like this to me, that the joy of riding was enhanced by the feeling that Malachy's pleasure must exceed mine. I could get from 'A' to 'B' by my own exertion if required, while he couldn't. It was Malachy time more so because the only reason I learnt to ride one of these was because he had brought the use for it into our life. As I turned the machine around to negotiate a gravelled practice circuit, I felt that closeness again, imagining the unburdening effect of its powered motion on my energy-limited son. In parallel I shared the excitement of competing with the others to circuit the track most skilfully, while also drifting into my private reminiscence.

The company hadn't had a tour group like us before, in which every member already had Segway skills, so the introduction was abbreviated, and we headed to the forest trails without some of the usual encumbrance. At our suggestion, the tour guide set out to go faster and further than usual.

As we skimmed along the trails, I found myself once more transported in time, to an earlier use of the Segway, feeling again the tremendous pleasure of flying along the White Sands Walk along the shores of Jervis Bay at sunset, my camera slung over my shoulder, on a lone search for the elusive perfect photo. The sensation was truly wonderful, allowing brisk travel between vantage points, with so little attention needed to steer or balance, and virtually no physical effort at all. It felt so contrary to intuition that such movement could cost me nothing in effort but produce a soothing rush of wind in my face, as the sound of the beach and the colours of a fading sun washed over me.

Segway riding was imbued with the memory of such untainted happiness, but also now with the sadness of grief. It was another face of the recurring grief paradox; the pain of remembrance brought me where I most wanted to be, close to Malachy.

Turning a corner in the trail with our guide, we struck a curiosity. Towering three tiers upward toward the foliage of the eucalypts was a pagoda-like building, each level smaller than the one below, each separated from the other by a glassed-in viewing platform. The unexpected feature was at once strangely out of place and a perfect photo opportunity. We spun our Segways into line in front of the building and modelled. Comfortable as we were with the devices, we were able to effect a hands-free, completely relaxed, 'playing it cool' pose for the camera.

I look at that photograph now and see a lifetime in that instant. There is the fun of that shared experience—adventurers in the forest, enjoying their riding skill, while pulling off the mock cool of the pouting model. Looking closely at the image uncovers also the strain of wanting to be happy as we are, while incomplete. We'd often before commented how quiet the house was when one of our four children was away. Five people seems a big family, but not when you started with six.

Maggie is thumbs-up at the left of the image, with effort putting a cheery smile in place, mirroring Seamus's expression at the opposite end, while the other three of us imitate Victorian era terseness in the middle. The family proudly, and with a hint of humour looks to the future, with a 'This Is Us Now' determination. Each of us in our own way is showing our will to go on, to suppress the agony of our disrupted life, to rediscover light in a world grown darker.

For all the trauma of our grief life did go on. By the time we reached home in Nowra, 2013 had become 2014. Imogen would resume her studies, combining Civil Engineering with an Arts degree, majoring in philosophy. Seamus, despite the ruin of his final months of school, did find a way into an undergraduate degree in Medicine. 'Following in Dad's footsteps' as some would assert to his feigned annoyance. Niamh had two years yet to run at Loreto, which provided a secure replacement for home.

That summer holiday in Tasmania did produce some moments of unblemished fun, of unselfconscious pleasure. Perhaps its lesson was that of keeping busy. Carry on doing things as you would if you were happy.

What we hoped for the future was that moments, then minutes, then who knows, maybe even days or weeks of pleasure would gradually outnumber the others.

I tried over and over again to capture the perfect family photograph on that trip, and many tragi-beautiful images emerged. 'This Is Us Now' is a necessary position to adopt, but inescapably a sad one. In a way we are no longer merely a family, we are defined by being the survivors in a family.

Music to grieve by

'This Is Us Now' felt important to assert. Maggie and I wanted Imogen, Seamus and Niamh to know they are enough for us, each worthy of a full quota of parental love.

Inescapably, every photo is incomplete. Every photo, like everything we do, has a Malachy-shaped shadow.

56

LIVING ON

Those words were pure freedom. They could only be written by someone who had already found himself in the third stage of life, when a person cease to minister to his immortality and no longer considers it a serious matter.

— Milan Kundera

After a longer than usual absence, the back gate swung open to admit a huffing, panting Maggie, on return from her run. Endorphins and solitude were her grief drug of choice. Breathing hard, I noted the fair skin of her arms was moist with sweat, her face drenched wet with tears. Running and crying, then crying some more, was becoming an established practice in the post-funeral 'let down' period.

Once she caught her breath, Maggie described the intense experience of her run, iPod strapped to her arm, a playlist of 'Malachy Music' was her companion on the road. The melody helps break down the tedium of the exercise, and the beat helps force the pace. Maggie stared at me and exclaimed, 'I know it's not real, but I swear Malachy is talking to me through the music'.

Distressing as it was, Maggie made a solid case linking the lyrics she described to our dead child. Something about the 'shuffle' function of an iPod sometimes fails to convince the songs appear completely at random. Granted the music was selected in keeping with Malachy's taste, but it felt with this as if he were determined to be reflected in every tune and every lyric.

The mourner's void was fast being filled by Malachy himself.

The dead man's tastes and interests were so broad it seemed he touched everything my mind turned to; every song I heard was either just his taste, or something he'd expressed a contrary view of, every news item seemed to involve something he'd been interested in. All of a sudden, every slice of Pop culture seemed to reference death, sick children, or child prodigiousness. While living, Malachy was larger than life, in death he was amplified all the more.

Numb to most things, and probably less aware than usual of my surrounds, I remember noticing a few things. I noticed Seamus was often missing from the public areas within the house, and that a search would find him alone, silent, in his brother's room, just lying on the bed. Just lying. No words required.

A paradox of grief became obvious. Sobbing and choking is horrible, and distressing. You can't feel any sadder than when those waves overwhelm you. On the other hand, when you feel at your most distressed, you also feel closer to the object of loss. The more acutely your grief is felt, the stronger and more tangible the emotional attachment.

I can understand people who don't want the grief to fade. We owe the loved one a debt of emotion, so to leave this behind can feel like failing in our obligation.

Pain is desirable because pain is closeness, and immediacy, and sharpens our memories.

Pain is undesirable because life must go on. Our family had to live on, without Malachy, but with, in his place, the void.

We would each wrestle with the tension of needing not to forget, but having to protect ourselves from pain, and each find a balance somewhere different. As time progressed, Maggie and Niamh leaned to frequent remembrance, Seamus and Imogen more toward trying to ignore the traumatic shadow. I was stranded somewhere between, alternately drawn to both options.

The Arctic Monkeys, about whom Mac had been fanatical, were coming to Sydney in May 2014. Having secured tickets and protected the date in our calendars, the upcoming concert became a fixed point in our grieving process. We all loved the band, no one more than Mac. Their latest album had become associated with Malachy's death after being the soundtrack of his final days. The concert would force our grief, our Malachy to the fore again. It had the potential to be cathartic having elements of 'reliving', being the epitome of 'Mac-Music' but also a chance to do some 'ignoring' style mourning, as the music is exhilarating in its own right.

As the date approached, we tried to make contact with the band, through Maggie's letter, to request a song dedication. Through circumstance we kept missing our target. By the time we walked in to join the crowd below the stage at Sydney's Entertainment Centre, we had no word as to whether the band had heard Maggie's plea.

We were aware that the concert had significance not only to us, but also to a wider circle of Malachy's survivors. The atmosphere was heavy with anticipation as we made our way into the throng on the floor in front of the stage. The support act was a smooth sounding band, including Tame Impala front man, Kevin Parker. The crowd moved happily in time to their ambient sound. Once they vacated the stage the crush was on. More and more people forced their way front and centre, in a pattern that continued through the Arctic Monkeys set. Our group was splintered, and we watched the children disappear sideways and backwards through the crowds as the surge of bodies dictated. Maggie and I both tried to resist the late invaders, as we wanted our early arrival to be rewarded by proximity to the stage. Being the oldest fans we encountered, seemed justification in itself for holding our ground.

We were hoping the band would be talkative, providing a chance for the hoped-for shoutout for Malachy. Lead singer, Alex Turner, is one of the foremost lyricists of the era, so the manner of banter he would provide was a matter of some interest. A couple of years earlier I had been entertained by an interview he gave to the Australian ABC radio station, Triple J. The density of Turner's Sheffield accent made him barely intelligible to the local presenters.

So bemused were they that they made a point of how hilarious it was; one of the chief wordsmiths of independent music could scarcely utter a word an Australian listener could decipher. The DJ turned it into a challenge to his audience, to phone in and translate the words of the young bard. A woman from Sheffield stepped in to save the day, explaining it was simple, 'What he said was "(string of unintelligible Sheffield accent…)".'

All we got from Alex was: 'Hello, Sydney. Great to see you again.'

Once the set was up and running it became clear the band's vibe was to let the music do the talking—idle fan chat between songs was completely absent. The show was a fantastic indie rock performance, not a fireside chat. It was brilliant. We bounced and cheered and sang along as one buzz followed another, the familiar pounding and reverberant rhythms, barking rhymes and smart lyrics commanded every space of the stadium.

By the time the Monkeys cranked out their smoother version of John Cooper Clarke's 1982 punk poetry classic *I Wanna Be Yours* as the second track of their encore, we knew the night had run its course. The audience had worked themselves to a lather and ridden the ups and downs of a beautifully constructed set list, leaning heavily on the current album, 'AM', but pumping up the ante with favourites from their back-catalogue. As Clarke's poem faded out, Alex ran through the parting formalities:

(My Translation) 'Thank you, Sydney. It's been an absolute pleasure to be back here. Thank you for havin' us …'

With a tiny bit more banter, Alex Turner's left hand raised part in greeting, part salute. He paused momentarily, then this:

'Thank you. Thank you so much. THIS ONE GOES OUT TO MALACHY. It's called, *ARE YOU MINE.*'

The last of this was nearly lost in the scream that emerged, unannounced, from my chest. I felt my throat sting with the strain of a prolonged ecstatic yell as my head filled with blood and months of empty despair burst from my body. The crowd bounced rhythmically as one, while the jarring crash of the guitars dictated our timing. The pent-up joy of the whole stadium found satisfaction in the rush of beautiful noise, though none but the knowing few could share the cathartic flood of emotion that swamped Maggie and me.

It is a moment forever fresh in memory. A tribute to the best, greatest, most loved son in Elysium, from the people he had proclaimed the best band in the world.

When the band left the stage for the last time and the lights came up, we loitered on the floor of the stadium, not wanting to let the moment recede. Promptly the floor emptied, except for a growing number of stragglers, drawn from the stalls and around the standing room. With everyone else gone, the dance floor housed a small crowd, a select group who knew the meaning of the final tribute.

Friends of ours, and friends of the children kept appearing from amongst the dispersing throng. We all shared the 'Wow' moment, stunned by the reminder of our lost boy. There was nothing much to say. In the end our motley gathering of Malachy-related loiterers, lost in reverie, was herded from the floor by the security staff.

57

WHAT GOES AND WHAT STAYS

Wherever he steps, whatever he touches, whatever he leaves,
even unconsciously, will serve as a silent witness...

— Paul L Kirk

One year after Malachy's death I took advantage of some time alone at home to steal into his room with my camera. In the immediate aftermath of his death Seamus had spent much time just being in the room. Everything about it resonated with the boys' shared history and the varied passions of the younger brother. The two boys had shared the bedroom for the years leading up to our Irish adventure.

The room housed Malachy's trove of precious artefacts, containing tiny clues to unveil parts of the child, and then the young man, that might otherwise slide through without notice. Cane baskets sit filled with haphazard piles of Mac's soft toys and figurines, a monument to their myriad of forgotten back stories, known only to their creator.

There are diaries and private notebooks, filling out the picture of Mac's life quietly blossoming under our unsuspecting noses. I had had secret moments in my life forging my future identity away from the reach of parents, friends, or siblings. With his death Malachy's room yields some of those moments in his life to the observer. Malachy loved to put his thoughts on paper. From time to time I leaf through the assorted documents that make up his writing legacy, including his reworking of the Max Martly script, and the unfinished story of Esteban Devereaux.

In the dark early days of mourning we had offered, and given away, various of Malachy's possessions to friends for whom they had meaning—ties and pens, the odd toy. We reasoned Malachy had no need of them and that storing his objects would do nothing to bring him back. I then spent a year having very mixed feelings about the room, which was largely left untouched. I would hurry past it on my way to or from the front door, afraid to face the inevitable flood of memories within.

After a year Maggie and I felt the room needed using as something other than a mausoleum. We decided one bedroom would become a guest room. Seamus was offered the choice to stay where he was, or to take possession of Mac's room.

Seamus chose to inherit his brother's space. So, the time came for the room to be cleared out. Irrational as it may seem, I feared I was losing something more of my son in the process. I took photo after photo. With my camera I would soften the blow, preserving forever the room as it was. Whatever of Malachy remained there I recorded. If we had to throw his stuff away, we could at least retain its image, and stifle the fear of forgetting.

Malachy had been physically consigned to the slow lane by his underpowered heart. He turned his languidness to advantage by becoming observant. The 'superpower' of keen observation was one of his concepts that invaded my thinking. Walking together, I would try to get inside his experience by consciously slowing myself to his speed and observing as intently as I could. Streets and the bush came alive with detail when I could allow myself to move into Mac's low gear.

Dr Joseph Bell is widely believed to have been the template on which Sherlock Holmes was based. Arthur Conan Doyle acknowledged this, and traces of the brilliant, animated lecturer and renowned occupational physician are hard to ignore in the fictional genius of Holmes. Dr Bell was reputed to be able to tell you exactly what somebody did for a living by the time they had sat down in his consulting room to present their ailment. A callus on the thumb may be a clue to repeated chafing of a craftsman on their tools, while muscled arms indicated the demands of manual labour, or a stain on the skin the exposure to a particular chemical. Dr Bell's medical skills were apparently brought to bear on the hunt for the infamous nineteenth century serial murderer, Jack the Ripper.

In this glorious tradition of medical genius applied to forensic thinking there was another man in the twentieth century known as 'France's Sherlock Holmes'. His name is Dr Edmond Locard.

Locard was a pioneer of forensic science, famous for his dissertations on the idea that 'Every contact leaves a trace'. His 'Theory of Exchange' holds that when two objects come in contact with each other, both will be altered. Each will both gain something from the other and leave something behind.

In Locard's world, the room into which I brought my camera must be swimming in traces of Malachy. I hardly know what I hoped to find in there, but I knew I couldn't bear to lose another trace of the person who had called it his bedroom.

Part voyeur, part forensic detective, part grieving father, I froze in the middle of the room, shocked by the familiarity. Everything remained carefully in its place. It was as if Malachy had just left for school. In a few hours he would labour up the short hill from the bus stop, dig his keys from his pocket, throw open the door, toss his bag to the ground and call out a greeting.

In the corner I photographed his drum set, surrounded by posters proclaiming the 'Eight Best Bands of ALL TIME'. Sitting atop of the floor-tom, neatly placed, ready for today's practice, were his demonstration CD, lesson book, and sticks. I photographed countless objects I'd grown to associate with Malachy: Ninja Turtles, spinning tops, Lego, his array of soft toys, all the players of his endless fantasy saga. There was a box labelled 'T.O.M, Malachy', residual of the drama activities he'd been involved in with the 'Tournament Of Minds'. Locard's ideas about traces were not merely obvious in this place, they were overwhelming.

Opening each drawer and cupboard, I peered inside and was struck by the presence of my son. Even his underwear had poignancy, being as it was many sizes smaller than average for his age. Every nook spoke of who Malachy had been or more painfully, who he might yet have become.

The collection of prized possessions that sat on his cupboard included 'Peli', a Pelican in a helicopter hat. 'Peli' had been Mac's first toy, being a gift from the Child Flight helicopter that had borne him to Sydney for the first of his intensive hospital stays. There too was a soccer ball signed by the members of a famous soccer team, a gift from an admirer in the HeartKids world, and a figurine from Hanoi's renowned puppet theatre. Pensively stooped, guarding the collection, his head bowed, his hands clasping a golden heart to his chest was a small wooden statuette of a boy. Symbolising, perhaps, a son's deep abiding love for his mother. A boy with a golden heart.

Every object seemed loved for its meaning to Malachy. The boy, and then the emerging man took no joy in ownership for its own sake. How fitting it seemed that he'd disavowed any inherent right to good fortune and adopted a world view in which wealth ought to be shared. Malachy had spoken of the mere accident of birth by which his malformation was manageable in affluent Australia but would have been promptly fatal in the developing world. Things were secondary to people.

Malachy's lack of material attachment to things rang truer than ever as I examined the sum-total of his possessions. Every single possession was now useless to a fault. If I hadn't previously understood this truism about death, it now stamped itself indelibly in my core: 'You can't take it with you'.

Looking again at the evocative statuette of the boy with the golden heart, in the stillness of the room I cried for my own golden-hearted boy, whose every trace spoke of humour and enthusiasm, of music, colour and life.

To the right of the sculpted boy, lying free on the white painted surface, was a curious object. A horseshoe, twisted to its current shape in the hands of a giant sensei, lay awkwardly, robbed of its useful structure, waiting to be reshaped by the pupil's hands. Malachy's hands.

I pondered the object as time stood still, a small frozen moment in remembrance of a life punctuated by larger ones. A sense of something distilled in me. My son was dead and would never complete the designated task. The twisted iron, never to be reshaped, would not be nailed to the hoof of a horse. Contrary to Locard, the horseshoe is poignant for the trace Malachy won't leave. It will stay as it is, an enduring symbol of what might have been.

58

CHARITY SWANSONG

A speech should not just be a sharing of information,
but a sharing of yourself.

— Ralph Archbold

At the George Street end of Martin Place, in the heart of the
Central Business District sits the magnificent sandstone façade
of Sydney's General Post Office. Nestled behind the geometrically
carved heritage stone is a stylish, grand hotel, The Westin. In late
August 2014 Maggie, Imogen, Seamus, Niamh and I donned fancy
suits and dresses to join the formal fun of the annual HeartKids
New South Wales Tiny Tickers Ball. The ball, whose origins were
in Nowra, in 2004, is the premier fundraising and social event in
the HeartKids calendar. It is a familiar and much-loved gathering
for us and many others. We have keenly anticipated the event
many times through the years, sometimes as organisers, sometimes
as guests, twice as speakers, or as parents of a speaker.

Dressed at our most splendid, that one day of the year, we meet
old friends, some of them colleagues in the pursuit of a better life
for our children, some doctors and nurses who care for Heart Kids,
some of them survivors or family members. In short, we spend the
evening with all manner of people who share a profound bond.
The ballroom fills with those who have felt the touch of childhood
heart disease, decked out in formal splendour, putting the happiest
possible face on their concern.

We attended as bereaved parents. I had a small role to play, with the organisation honouring me with award of life membership, recognising what the inscription describes as my 'significant contribution to HeartKids NSW'.

Maggie had the more challenging role: to deliver the parent testimonial. Typically, a touching story from the mother of a Heart Kid, about their plight, and the struggles faced by the family, ultimately reinforcing the worthiness of the cause, before the charity auction launches. We had each been part of this before, but not as parents of a dead boy.

Maggie now had the same mixed sense of fear and opportunity stalking her through the lead-up to this ball as I had previously had for Malachy's funeral. Balancing the awful sadness of grief, that thing all 'heart-parents' most fear, against the hope of something better was critical to the success of this address. To ignore the depth of her sorrow would be false, but too much sorrow or despair does not make for happy donors.

Maggie's tragedy was well enough known to many of the five hundred-strong crowd. How she might weave a thread of hope and joy into the narrative was known only to her.

Professional as always, Maggie had put together a range of slides to be projected to the large screens behind her at points in the speech. I made my way to the back of the hall, adjacent to the projectionist, to help out should confusion arise in the job.

As the MC introduced Maggie many held their breath. A hush blanketed the room. My heart was in my mouth, seized with apprehension. Slender in orange and pink, Maggie stepped to the lectern. The fine tremor of her limbs scarcely detectable, she radiated maternal calm as she softly cleared her voice, before taking one long measured breath, and opening:

This one goes out to Malachy. Leonard Cohen's poem 'Anthem' repeats the following verse:

Ring the bells that still can ring, forget your perfect offering.

> There is a crack, a crack in everything, that's how
> the light gets in.

This stanza expresses the conviction that even in the darkest moments of our lives, somewhere, through a crack, a ray of light and hope can enter. My personal testament as a parent of a child with heart disease is in some ways a tale of darkness, sadness and loss but I want to tell you also how Malachy and HeartKids provided a ray of light and beacon of hope through the many challenges we faced.

An effective debater in her school days, and competent presenter through her working life, Maggie paced herself steadily, gradually showing her audience the risk of a weeping meltdown into incoherence was not to be realised that night.

The timing of Malachy's fatal collapse, just two days after that ball was revealed to the audience. Maggie continued, after describing the drama of the collapse, the failed resuscitation, and the helicopter ride to Westmead that fateful day:

> Children's Hospital Westmead is unfortunately a place that we have spent too much time as a family over the years. However, that evening I was relieved to be back and hopeful that Malachy would recover from this serious incident as he had done so many times before. It was clearly a grave concern, given Malachy's history, that an arrest outside of a hospital, with such a long resuscitation carried a high risk of serious brain damage. Malachy never woke up and died in ICU with his brother Seamus, sisters Imogen and Niamh, Dom and I by his side. Malachy was cared for wonderfully, to a natural death surrounded by the people he loved.

Maggie explained her inspiration to sign up to the HeartKids cause. The better-known Heart Foundation, she would discover, really wasn't interested in children, its primary concerns were problems of ageing. Maggie was determined to find a better future.

In the time of darkness HeartKids was that ray of light. After hearing of HeartKids, I remember deciding that it would be excellent therapy for me to get involved in the cause of Childhood Heart Disease and help raise money specifically for children's heart research. I felt inspired to know there might be a way I could help my son, and others like him. Malachy's condition was fraught with complications, so much so that we have not always had full agreement between the professionals involved in his care. At times this added stress and made our decisions about Malachy's care even more difficult. The general public has limited awareness of the seriousness of some children's conditions. I often had to suffer people's well-meaning opinions about how amazing medical technology is today and how sure we can be Malachy will be cured. Well, it is in some ways amazing, but for Malachy that cure never came. The more I learnt, the more gaps I discovered in services and treatment for these medically challenged children.

The audience did not stir as Maggie described her early involvement, with the 'Malachy and Friends Ball' in Nowra, and the emergence of Malachy's pride in being a HeartKid, and the pleasure he took from knowing there was an organisation that held his needs and those of his affected friends foremost in its ambitions.

Drawing attention to the screen behind her, Maggie invited people to watch a video of that show-stopping moment from the 2011 ball. Many had seen it live, but the impact had not diminished, as the diminutive 12-year-old paused before declaring, 'I'm proud of being blue'. HeartKids was indeed something of a saviour to us:

Malachy (and his siblings) loved the Christmas parties, the family camps and indeed Malachy had wonderful enriching experiences at two Teen camps. He made some great friends and we remember him really deeply analysing how interesting it was to meet kids like himself who actually understood him and had such similar experiences to him.

Maggie spoke of Malachy's nature, and the maturing effect of his disease:

> Malachy was wise beyond his years, I guess this came partly from his illness and the constant pressure of learning how to adjust to an unusual life, different from his peers and siblings. He had faced death several times, some he could remember and some he could not. He had many nightmares about death and really had to come to grips with his own mortality in a way that most people don't need to. Malachy had told us what song he wanted played at his funeral and he even had instructed me to tell Dom to 'crack a few gags' during his eulogy as he wanted us to be happy when we thought of him. He was a boy of many interests a comedian, a writer, a film director. I was reading over his last story he wrote recently and wanted to share the unique way he even actually personified death in one of his stories—it went like this...
>
> > 'Oh, hey death, listen man I'm good why don't you just go back to your wife and kids I'll be fine don't you worry just come back for me in seventy years' time!'
>
> Malachy wrote that profound message to death only one month before he died. It is absolutely heart-breaking having to talk to your child about death and I was always quietly reassuring him that he would be fine, even though I understood and shared his fear.

Maggie paid additional tribute to the siblings of our now immortal son, and hopefully in so doing helped other siblings be less forgotten. The degree to which Malachy's illness and disability drew us away from our other children is hard to measure. It was even harder to avoid, with his needs being so immediate, and the stakes so high. They must carry some of the scars of his neediness:

> Malachy was lucky to have older siblings who treated him like a normal little boy. Dressing him up as a little girl, stuffing him in boxes, teasing him, sharing so much fun and mischief and making sure he knew he was not any more special than

them. I am so amazingly proud of my children and grateful for how much value, fun and interest they added to his short life. I know it is hard being the sibling of a sick child because at times you miss out and get ignored and probably feel like mum or dad don't worry about you as much as the 'sick one' but mostly because you have to grow up and live your adult life without your childhood friend and brother.

Tears of recognition ran down Imogen's face. Each of our surviving children had at times been neglected by necessity, but not ever for one second unloved or forgotten.

Maggie drew to her conclusion:

'There is a crack, a crack in everything,
That's how the light gets in.'

Malachy, you are an inspiration to so many, you lived your life to the full, you were a ray of sunshine. I am honoured to be your mum and I miss you so much.

The blanket of hush drew closer as people drew breath. To a person we absorbed the sobering depth of the parenting journey this most beautiful of women had endured. Silently, we admired the bravery and steadiness with which she bared her soul for the audience. The echoing 'clack', 'clack', 'clack' of her heels down the steps from the podium rang out across the silence. The spell of quietude was broken, and applause filled the hall, following Maggie back to her seat where she was greeted by the hugs of her grown children.

59

A LIGHT ON A HILL

When you take a flower in your hand and really look at it, it's your world for the moment. I want to give that world to someone else.

— Georgia O'Keeffe

Malachy's 17th birthday came towards the end of the longest warm spell in the history of local weather records. By mid-morning the leaf-filtered sunlight reaching our back garden was warm enough to induce a light sweat as I descended the stairs from the veranda. I wore my brown bushman style hat, in habitual deference to the sun's ability to penetrate and burn my fair Irish skin.

The day was quiet and still, with nothing to threaten the comforting solitude of the garden. It suited me to be alone with my thoughts. Memories of happier birthdays bubbled chaotically under my calm exterior. The dead calm of grief held me still. Grief creates an intuitive straightjacket; the noisier and stronger the emotion, the more the demand for silence. I felt that to speak, or break my silence, would unleash a flood of unwanted emotion. As long as I stayed silent the brittle wall holding my grief in check would hold. In silence the sun would warm and cheer me.

The soothing heat of the sun is timeless. In its embrace, with my eyes closed, I imagined myself back into childhood. Before the age of doubt and disappointment, and the tragedy of maternal sickness, before first knowing failure. Back I travelled to a time before love and marriage, before work and children, back in short to a time before Malachy's death. As the sun warmed deeper into my back and shoulders, through into the bones of my arms as I tended the garden, I drifted back to a time when Malachy was alive.

Secateurs in hand I walked the garden with Malachy. He was almost tangible as I searched for fresh blooms. Mauves and pinks were in bloom as I reached to prune the colourful tips from the crepe myrtle. Walking to the shaded lower tier of the garden I felt and heard the light crunch of crushed granite beneath my feet. I strode to the very bottom corner, where a weeping maple dragged its skirt on the moist earth. We'd planted it six months earlier, on the anniversary of Malachy's death. The commemorative plant surrendered two fronds to my pruning tool. I mentally noted, to Malachy and for my own comfort, the beauty of the filigreed purple leaves.

Moving around the garden, cane basket in hand, I built a pile of plant matter, with any flowers whose display caught my eye, and foliage of various shades. I sank into mindfulness as butterflies wafted in and out of view, and birds played in branches above. I felt the tension down my arm into my right hand as I squeezed the handles of the secateurs, slicing through branches of native Lilli Pilli, fresh sprouts of Murraya and a flowering shrub behind our front fence.

An internal dialogue of memories, of Malachy and of a time before Malachy continued back and forward inside my head. Nothing was concluded. No coherent ideas emerged, but the longer I walked in silence and pruned the steadier I felt.

The basket filled and I returned to the back veranda. I placed the secateurs I had used and a spare set into the basket and concluded my reverie.

'Maggie, are you ready?' I called.

'Yep, let's go,' came back from the study.

With unspoken reverence each for the other's wounded heart, we drove through town, then headed east towards Greenwell Point.

Turning right at the Worrigee Road, we swung into a side street to pick up Malachy's oldest friend, Ryan. Loyal beyond death, Ryan had taken the day off school, and was home alone while his parents worked. Sombre greetings showed deference to the occasion.

Three of us now, quiet within the car, we made our way past the rural properties, blocks of several acres, perfect for horse lovers. We drove past lightly wooded eucalypt forests and a familiar reception centre, until we reached our destination. Removing the basket from the back seat we made the short walk in silence, stopping just short of the sandstone boulder that now represents the life that was Malachy.

Sprigs of fresh flowers from an unknown garden sat upright in the vases beside Malachy's boulder, along with two potted fuchsias, one to either side. Some cacti and a small shaggy teddy sat in front. The dried remains of the last batch of flowers we'd placed sat relieved of their petals in the last of the water, now darkened by the decomposing stems. Wordlessly I removed the moulding matter from the vases, spreading it on the forest floor to let nature reclaim its own. Maggie, becalmed in her grief, watched from a few feet away as I gathered the empty vases and walked off to a nearby tap to refill them. Ryan silently nursed the pain of his own loss.

The lawn cemetery provides water receptacles with a spike protruding from the base, allowing mourners to spear as many as needed into the ground without need for propping up. I methodically filled each vase in turn, spiking them into the ground behind the tap.

I returned with my fresh water supply, implanting the vases in the soil surrounding Malachy's rock. Maggie and I distributed our stock of flowers and foliage evenly between several vases, which we arranged for maximum aesthetic appeal. Strips of bark and fallen branches from the surrounding trees lay haphazardly around the site. I found perverse pleasure in moving these, tending the site to neatness. Small gentle placements of leaf matter, twigs and flakes of bark felt significant to me. The tenderness of this ritual was somehow comforting. My body had a reason to move while unseen tears fell into the frame of my sunglasses. Tidying and beautifying this tiny patch of mother earth was not in itself enough reason to be at this place, at this time.

I know tidying up is not why Maggie, Ryan and I are here. I know we are here because Malachy is dead. Two and a half years dead. Malachy's ashes lie here, sealed and buried in a blue plastic container. Meticulous gardening is a futile expression of care for my child. Malachy lies beyond the need for any such tenderness.

As if straightening my son's tie on the way out the door for his first day of school, I moved aside nature's mess, and tended our cut offerings into the desired form. The heat of the day was not yet at its peak. It would reach thirty-one degrees that autumn day. A faint breeze left a coolness down the tracks of my tears.

Six vases of flowers were spiked into the earth, and the blooms and foliage teased into a balanced display, with colour and greenery evenly spread around the symbolic stone. The shaggy little bear was adjusted to sit modestly in the miniature forest. I fluffed its fur to reverse the grooming effect of the last rainfall before placing him back at his post. A frond of Malachy's weeping maple was the last piece to be moved into place, its stem lightly resting on the top of the stone, with a leafy tendril reaching downwards to the edge of the inlaid plaque.

That composition on the plaque dated back to those darkest of days, after Malachy had died, but before his formal farewell. Together the five of us had laughed about all the ways he either defined himself, or was labelled by us, and collaborated to write a notice that would end up reflected in the text of his gravestone.

MALACHY DECLAN MANDELA FRAWLEY

2ND MARCH 1999 ~ 9TH SEPTEMBER 2013

RACONTEUR, AUTHOR, COMEDIAN, DRUMMER, FILM DIRECTOR,
HEART KID, TIE-WEARING SON, BROTHER AND FRIEND

MALACHY INSPIRED WITH HIS COURAGE AND RESILIENCE
HE ENGAGED PEOPLE WITH COMPASSION, WIT AND ENTHUSIASM

'MAC' IS DEEPLY LOVED BY MANY WHO SHARED HIS PATH
HE IS TREASURED BY THE FRAWLEY AND NOBLE FAMILIES

MALACHY IS ESPECIALLY MISSED AND CELEBRATED BY
IMOGEN, SEAMUS, NIAMH, MAGGIE AND DOM

Staring at Malachy's rock, with a familiar moisture catching in the rims of my sunglasses part of me wanted to stay there forever, the closest I can get to Mac. The first to break the silence with a move towards the car would implicitly put pressure on the others to follow, but I sensed if no one moved we could be stuck there endlessly. At some point I broke the trance, reluctantly drifting back in the direction of the gate. Maggie and Ryan followed in the quiet, the only sound was the light crunch of our feet on the gravel.

Once back in the car, leaving the cemetery, we sounded Ryan out regarding his plans for the day, which it turned out were mainly to be at home with his grief, so we brought him in on the next leg of our journey. Destination Kangaroo Valley.

The trip was very familiar to Maggie and me. At a fairly young age the children had developed a love of a Sunday ritual of driving to Kangaroo Valley, stopping for Mass at St Joseph's church, then browsing the heritage town. The church is perched uphill from the road, modestly shrouded in forest. It has been steadily restored through the efforts of priest and congregation over the twenty years we've known it. Its stained-glass windows have been replaced and modernised one by one over this time, putting a fresh face on the historical beauty of this form of religious art. The local priest was a hermit, Father Ronan, known for his sonorous lilting sermons, which on one occasion left Niamh and Malachy distracted enough to secretly etch their initials on the back of the third pew. After Father Ronan's Baroque-style mass, replete with frankincense and Gregorian intonations, it was our custom to visit a lolly store, then a pie shop or café, and enjoy a lunch on the town.

Maggie and I had both wanted to come here on this day. Not just for the calm it bestowed, and its place in our domestic history, but also because of a project we'd heard was afoot. PJ's grandmother Anne was Father Ronan's loyal aide and had explained that the last of the leadlight windows, being fashioned in Europe, was being funded by a bequest. The family of the donor did not wish to be acknowledged in the accompanying dedication. The window was to depict St Monica, the patron saint of mothers. The benefactors asked the parish community to instead use the name of a member of the local congregation. A child, representing maternal care and love for children, would be named on the plaque. Anne's suggestion that Malachy be that child had been approved.

Recently having heard that the finished window was being shipped to Australia, it occurred to Maggie and I to check on its progress.

We parked on the road below and looked uphill at the church. With some trepidation we made the short climb to the entrance vestibule. We felt touched that Mac would be officially remembered here, carrying our secret knowledge of the mark he'd already left on the pew. We intuited there would be some solace in this peaceful hideaway. Hearts heavy, we pushed on the tall double doors. To no effect. Unyielding. Locked! Darn, there goes the plan.

As I backed a little down the hill, I felt the futility of it all. All the build-up to a flop, and an impotent struggle to even enter the church. The weight of quiet inside an empty church still has a calming power for me, despite scepticism's grip on my rational mind. But it wasn't to be.

Or was it?

Though reluctant to interrupt the cloistered serenity within, I desperately wanted our pilgrimage to have an outcome other than simply fizzling out. While wrestling between retreat and pursuit I wandered up a narrow bush path to the left of the church. This led under a bower of flowering vines to a timber gate, the boundary between the Hermit life and the world at large. I searched for a bell or buzzer, hoping there was a designated way to gain attention.

Raising my eyes to the right, I spied a bell with a short rope, and sought Maggie's approval to tug for attention. Reaching, I noticed something. Behind and above the bell was the rearmost window on that side of the church, the back-left panel, due to be last renovated. A shaft of Autumn sunlight reflected from the newly installed panes, which struck me at once with their beauty. My heart skipped as it dawned on me what I was looking at. Beneath the majestic arched window was a smaller, square panel, where I could make out, reversed, the text of my son's name.

$$\boxed{\text{YHƆAlAM}}$$

I rang the bell, as Maggie, Ryan and I stared at the window, hoping there'd be an answer. And there was. The gate swung open. Ronan, traditional monk's habit flowing to the ground, flashed an angelic grin, and greeted us warmly, waving us through. We followed along the side path and into the sacred quiet of the church.

I trod lightly, in cautious reverence toward the sunlit rear window. Ronan reported that by good fortune the window had arrived sooner than expected and described the symbolic content of the work. This included the legend that recalls St Monica crying before God every night in the hope of seeing the reform of her wayward son, Augustine, who duly reformed to become one of the most exalted of the Roman Catholic saints. Father Ronan slipped away, leaving us space for contemplation.

Sure enough, Monica, her shoulders brightest as the sun bore through them at that time of day, had her head bowed in sorrow. Tenderly she yearns for the safety and maturation of her beloved son.

Craving solitude to nurse the rising flood of my emotion, I drifted to sit in the familiarity of Pew Three and touched the fading scratch marks made in life by my own son, whose safe maturation would never be realised. I kept still, seeking to master enough calm indifference to keep soaking in the sad beauty of another frozen moment.

Moving back into the light passing through St Monica, I pondered the love I felt, the painful aching exaltation at having another place to be close to Malachy. In a rush so much of life, so many moments coalesced to bring the essence of our child to the fore. In that moment I understood Monica, and every parent forced to fear for the child they love. As the autumn sun pushed its warm consolation through the tinted glass I understood the depth of joy my child had brought to me, and his capacity to reach into the hearts of others. I felt again the depth and breadth of grief.

I had arrived expecting to hear of a plaque yet to bear Malachy's name, but as I stared ahead through the backlit inscription of the square window beneath the feet of the saint, the sun amplified a phrase on the lower pane. I felt Malachy, always tugging at the hearts of people in life, now laid in the earth as ash, reaching beyond death to touch his grieving father. Perhaps this is why we live on, hoping and fighting for a better world. Here Malachy, in one phrase, made radiant by the distant sun, is immortalised. The phrase reflects my inspiration to share our story.

FOR
MALACHY
& ALL OUR
CHILDREN

ACKNOWLEDGEMENTS

There are two types of acknowledgements I'd like to make with respect to Malachy's story: those who carried us in life and those who carried the story to the page.

Firstly, I recognise what tremendous cooperative work went into making Malachy's life the joyous and fruitful adventure it proved to be.

To that end I owe everything to Maggie, Imogen, Seamus, Niamh and Malachy, who have brought happiness beyond any foreseen future. We have all been supported by a wide circle of friends and family who bought into the project of making Malachy's life what it became.

The town of Nowra rallied around us after Malachy's birth, in the process transforming from a nice place to work to a home for life. The school communities of St Michael's and St John's were key supports throughout, as were my colleagues and staff in general practice.

Special thanks to Colleen Mackey who loved the little Frawleys when their parents weren't around, and Malachy's friends, in particular Ryan and PJ with whom he spent so much of his time. This also involved lots of care from their parents, Terry and Donna, Paul and Jeanna.

Thanks also to Duane, whose mentorship of Malachy included looking out for Maggie and me.

HeartKids was instrumental in turning our personal distress into a rallying cry and a force for good. We are forever in solidarity with their cause, and especially those who shared our passion to grow the work of the organisation. This includes Neil McWhannell, Lee Morgan, Rowena Whewell, Ryan Payne, Peter and Karen

Acknowledgements

Sherlock, Dawn Everingham, Mary Bowie, Stephen Shepherd, Cecily Waterworth, Alison Byrne, Simon Reeve and numerous others.

For the life-saving heroics and all manner of other care: we are grateful to the nursing staff, social workers, doctors and others we encountered at Sydney Children's Hospital Randwick, and The Children's Hospital Westmead, as well as the Children's Heart Research Centre for their ongoing search for useful knowledge. Foremost among these are Malachy's cardiologists, Garry Sholler and Stephen Cooper, and his surgeons, Graham Nunn, Richard Chard, and David Winlaw.

Some light was also brought into our lives by the wonderful people at Ronald McDonald House facilities at both Randwick and Westmead, and all associated with Make-A-Wish Australia.

When it comes to the writing of *Malachy* I must thank all at Junction Street Family Practice, who covered my intermittent absences to record this story. This was mostly done over the two-year period from June 2014 to June 2016.

Foremost Maggie, who was consulted most steps along the way, and often arrived home to find me typing away intently, absorbed in reliving the multiple traumas that resurfaced day to day in the process of writing. What appears as strength in me has often depended on her steadfastness at my side.

Many thanks to early readers, Angela Lloyd, Cindy Pan, Vanessa O'Keefe and Sally Gaven, whose encouragement proved invaluable, and preserved my belief in the potential of Malachy's story to be meaningful to others.

To Bert Hingley whose review of the manuscript helped focus me, along with Cheryl Sawyer who inspired with her seafood paella as much as her many published works.

Thanks to Moira Downes at Dymocks, whose advice and guidance included helpful input from Yvette Gilfillan, as well as introducing me to Allison Tait. Allison's support and guidance has been tremendous, helping me understand the patience required in dealing with the publishing process, as well as warning of the subsequent challenges of professional authorship.

Thanks also to Jayne Blake and Melinda Tognini, from the HeartKids network, whose input led me to try my hand with Wild Dingo Press.

Glenda Downing was a wonderful structural editor for me, seeming to really understand the tone I was after, and encouraging a sense of timeline, which helped the story tell itself more coherently. Glenda's considered attention allowed me to let go of chapters once held dear.

Catherine Lewis at Wild Dingo Press has borne me safely through the editing process, winning me over or pushing me ahead as circumstance required. Her team has been swift and professional and always a pleasure to deal with. I am very grateful for their skill and judgment in bringing *Malachy* to its readers.

Malachy himself was a great inspiration for me when it came to writing. Shaping the story around a snippet of his writing in this memoir was something of a passion project. In bringing my reflections to the page one of my goals was to see Malachy attain his desire to have his work published while young. By serendipity his writing mirrors his personal journey, and he remains forever young.